The New Safeguarding Lead.
By Paul M. Armstrong.

First Edition - Published 2024

To Debra.

My friend, mentor and to whom I owe so very much.

Introduction.

If you had approached me two decades ago and told me that I would one day have the privilege of being a safeguarding officer I would have likely raised an eyebrow in bewilderment. The notion of undertaking such a role was nowhere on my radar at that time. It wasn't until much later in my professional journey that I serendipitously stumbled upon the path leading me into the realm of safeguarding as a career.

I started my journey with a national youth development organisation, where in my initial weeks, we underwent various training sessions, one of which focused on safeguarding. Strangely enough, something about that particular session resonated deeply within me, though I couldn't quite pinpoint what it was. Perhaps it was the skill and passion of the trainer, who later became not only a close friend but also a valued mentor. It was after this session that a realisation dawned on me. Here was an opportunity to truly make a meaningful impact. Driven by this newfound sense of purpose, I delved deeper into the realm of safeguarding. I sought out formal training and pursued qualifications in the field. Before long, I found myself stepping into my first safeguarding role, which involved handling cases and facilitating training sessions. Yet, with each passing day, my ambition grew, alongside my growing knowledge and expertise.

Fast forward to the present moment, and I find myself in the esteemed position of lead safeguarding officer for a prominent UK charity, highly regarded within the sector. And you know something? My passion for what I do remains as fervent as ever! Each day presents new challenges and opportunities, allowing me to share my expertise and promote best practices among a diverse array of individuals.

This book is written primarily as a trusted guide and ally for newly qualified safeguarding leads, offering invaluable insights and support as they navigate their roles. However, it is also designed to serve as a robust reference manual for seasoned officers seeking to deepen their understanding and refine their practices. I take immense pride in my work within the field of safeguarding, and it is my earnest desire that my unwavering passion shines through in the pages that follow.

Paul M. Armstrong
2024

PART ONE

UNDERSTANDING SAFEGUARDING

The role of the safeguarding lead

In purely simplistic terms, safeguarding refers to the measures taken to protect the health, well-being, and human rights of individuals, particularly those who are vulnerable to abuse, neglect, or exploitation. Safeguarding encompasses various aspects, including child protection, adult safeguarding, and safeguarding within specific sectors such as education, healthcare, social care, and voluntary organisations.

Broadly speaking, safeguarding applies to anyone who may be at risk of harm, and safeguarding at work is everyone's responsibility.

- Safeguarding children is a priority in the UK, with specific legislation such as the Children Act 1989 and the Children Act 2004 outlining the duties of local authorities and other agencies to ensure the welfare of children.

- Adults at Risk are adults who may be vulnerable due to age, disability, illness, or other factors. The Care Act 2014 sets out statutory guidance for local authorities on safeguarding adults at risk of abuse or neglect.

- Organisations have a duty of care to safeguard their employees and volunteers from harm, including risks such as discrimination, harassment, and exploitation in the workplace.

- Individuals accessing services such as healthcare, social care, education, and housing are entitled to be safeguarded from harm while receiving support and assistance.

- Safeguarding also extends to the wider community, with efforts to prevent and address issues such as domestic violence, radicalisation, and online exploitation.

- Safeguarding responsibilities are shared among various agencies, including local authorities, health and social care services, educational institutions, law enforcement agencies, and voluntary organisations. Each sector has its own specific safeguarding policies, procedures, and guidelines tailored to the needs of the individuals they serve. Ultimately. safeguarding is a collective effort involving collaboration, vigilance, and commitment to promoting the safety and well-being of all individuals, particularly those who are most vulnerable.

- Being a safeguarding lead is a significant responsibility with far-reaching implications. At its core, the role involves being the primary point of contact and coordination for all safeguarding matters within an organisation or community. This entails several key responsibilities

- Safeguarding leads are responsible for implementing and ensuring compliance with safeguarding policies and procedures. This involves developing clear guidelines, disseminating information, and overseeing adherence to established protocols.

- Identifying and assessing potential risks to vulnerable individuals is a critical aspect of the role. Safeguarding leads must be vigilant in recognising signs of abuse or neglect and taking appropriate action to mitigate these risks.

- Educating staff, volunteers, and other stakeholders on safeguarding principles and practices is essential. Safeguarding leads often organise training sessions, workshops, and awareness campaigns to promote a culture of vigilance and accountability.

- In the event of safeguarding concerns or incidents, the lead is responsible for coordinating an effective response. This may involve conducting investigations, making referrals to relevant authorities or support services, and ensuring accurate and timely reporting.

- Safeguarding leads often collaborate with external agencies, such as social services, the police service, schools and healthcare professionals, to ensure a coordinated response to safeguarding issues. Building strong networks and partnerships is crucial for effectively safeguarding vulnerable individuals.

We will expand on each of these points as we continue through this guide.

The five 'R's of safeguarding

In safeguarding discussions, the concept of the 5 'Rs' serves as a cornerstone, providing a framework for understanding and implementing effective safeguarding practices. Safeguarding leads play a pivotal role in ensuring a comprehensive understanding of each 'R' among their team members, thus embedding it into their training programs.

The 5 'Rs' of Safeguarding encompass a range of principles essential for safeguarding effectiveness:

- **RECOGNISE** - This references the ability to recognise signs and indicators of abuse, neglect, or harm across various contexts and demographics. By developing a keen eye for identifying potential risks and vulnerabilities, safeguarding leads empower their team members to intervene early and appropriately.

- **RESPOND** - A prompt and appropriate response is crucial when safeguarding concerns arise. Safeguarding leads must equip staff with the knowledge and skills to respond effectively to disclosures, suspicions, or incidents of abuse, ensuring that individuals at risk receive the support and protection they need.

- **REPORT -** Timely and accurate reporting is fundamental for safeguarding accountability and intervention. Safeguarding leads must emphasise the importance of reporting concerns through the appropriate channels, whether internal reporting mechanisms or external agencies, and ensure staff understand their legal obligations and responsibilities in this regard.

- **RECORD** - Accurate and comprehensive record-keeping is essential for documenting safeguarding concerns, actions taken, and outcomes. Safeguarding leads should emphasise the importance of maintaining detailed records, ensuring transparency, accountability, and continuity of care for individuals involved in safeguarding processes.

- **REFER** - Continuous review and evaluation are essential for enhancing safeguarding practices and addressing any gaps or areas for improvement. Safeguarding leads should encourage a culture of reflection and learning within their teams, facilitating regular reviews of safeguarding procedures, policies, and training programs to ensure they remain relevant and effective.

By instilling a thorough understanding of the 5 'Rs' into their training programs, safeguarding leads empower their workforce to uphold the highest standards of safeguarding practice, ultimately contributing to the safety and well-being of vulnerable individuals within their care.

The '2P' principal

I developed this principle as a foundational concept for the safeguarding training sessions I run. The reason behind its inclusion stems from my belief that it serves as a valuable tool for simplifying the distinctions between safeguarding children and safeguarding adults.

Safeguarding children is **PARAMOUNT**
Safeguarding adults is **PROPORTIONATE**

Let's break that down a little. When it comes to safeguarding children, it's crucial to uphold the primary principle outlined in the Children Act - that the welfare of the child is paramount. This principle encompasses several key considerations for safeguarders. Firstly, it means that we're not as constrained by professional restraint as we are when safeguarding adults. When we possess evidence or hold suspicions of abuse or neglect concerning children, we are empowered to report these concerns confidentially to the appropriate agencies without the necessity of seeking prior authorization. This autonomy enables swift and decisive action to safeguard the welfare of vulnerable children, ensuring that their well-being remains paramount.

We must also take into account the second principle of the Children Act, which emphasises the importance of taking timely and appropriate action. Failing to do so could potentially harm the child's welfare or compromise their living situation. Therefore, it is imperative that safeguarding actions are executed promptly and with due diligence to ensure the well-being of the child is safeguarded effectively.

On the other flip-side of this, when it comes to safeguarding adults, our approach must be proportionate and respectful of individual autonomy. In most instances, we operate under the principle of obtaining permission from the adult at risk before sharing information. We prioritise involving the adult in primary decision-making processes, ensuring that any measures implemented are tailored to their specific needs and focused on achieving positive outcomes. Additionally, it's important to recognize and respect an individual's right to make decisions that we or others may perceive as unwise. Later in this book, we will delve into the topic of mental capacity in greater detail.

Legal Framework

The current legal framework that is in place for the governance of safeguarding in the United Kingdom is both comprehensive and multifaceted. It encompasses various laws, regulations, and guidance documents across different jurisdictions and industry sectors.

For us to fully understand this broad spectrum we must begin by looking at the various pieces of legislation that apply to safeguarding.

<u>**Children**</u>

The central piece of legislation governing child safeguarding is undeniably the Children Act, an Act of Parliament that holds pivotal significance in safeguarding practices concerning children.

The Children Act has a rich history dating back to its inception in 1989. Prior to this landmark legislation, child welfare laws in the UK were scattered across various statutes, resulting in a fragmented and inconsistent approach to child protection.

The need for a comprehensive and unified legal framework became increasingly evident in the 1980s, amidst growing concerns about child abuse, neglect, and inadequate support for vulnerable children and families. The tragic deaths of children such as Jasmine Beckford and Kimberley Carlile underscored the urgent need for reform.

In response to these challenges, the **Children Act 1989** was introduced, representing a significant milestone in child welfare legislation. The Act aimed to prioritise the welfare of children above all else, establishing a clear set of principles to guide decision-making and intervention in cases involving children and families.

Key provisions of the Children Act 1989 are:

The welfare of the child is paramount. The Act enshrined this principle, meaning that any decisions or actions concerning a child must prioritise their best interests above all other considerations.

Delay is likely to prejudice the welfare of the child. Any postponement or hesitation in taking action to safeguard the child's well-being could have detrimental effects on their welfare. This provision emphasises the importance of swift and decisive intervention in situations where a child is at risk of harm or neglect. It underscores the urgency of prioritising the child's best interests and ensuring that necessary steps are taken promptly to protect them from harm and promote their welfare.

The "No Order" principle. This refers to the guiding principle that the court should refrain from making an order regarding a child unless it is necessary to do so. This principle stresses the importance of minimising state intervention in family matters and prioritising the preservation of familial relationships where possible. It remains the belief that the child will always be better kept within the family unit unless it is genuinely unsafe or detrimental to the child for a court to make an order otherwise. Keeping this at the forefront of their decision-making, the court considers whether making an order would genuinely benefit the child's welfare. If it determines that the child's welfare can be adequately safeguarded without the need for a formal court order, then no order should be made. Instead, the court may opt for less intrusive measures, such as providing advice, assistance, or support to the family, to address any concerns and promote the child's well-being.

Parental responsibility. The Act introduced the concept of parental responsibility, defining the rights, duties, powers, and responsibilities that parents have in relation to their children. This includes the responsibility to provide a safe and nurturing environment for their children.

Local Authority Duties. Local authorities were given specific duties and powers to safeguard and promote the welfare of children in their area. This included the establishment of Local Authority Children's Services departments responsible for providing support and intervention for vulnerable children and families.

Care Proceedings and Orders. The Act introduced a framework for care proceedings and court orders to protect children at risk of significant harm. This included provisions for emergency protection orders, care orders, and supervision orders, among others.

Since its enactment, the Children Act 1989 has been supplemented by subsequent legislation and amendments, including the **Children Act 2004**, which introduced further reforms to improve outcomes for children and strengthen safeguarding practices.

The 2004 act built upon the solid foundations of the 1988 act and introduced significant reforms aimed at improving outcomes for children and strengthening safeguarding practices. Additions include:

Every Child Matters. One of the central features of the Children Act 2004 is the introduction of the Every Child Matters framework. This framework outlines five key outcomes that are essential for children's well-being: being healthy, staying safe, enjoying and achieving, making a positive contribution, and achieving economic well-being. The Act places a duty on relevant agencies to work together to promote these outcomes for all children.;

Local Safeguarding Children Boards (LSCBs). The Children Act 2004 strengthens the role of LSCBs, which were first established under the Children Act 1989. These are multi-agency partnerships responsible for coordinating local efforts to safeguard and promote the welfare of children. The Act clarifies the functions and responsibilities of LSCBs and requires them to develop and implement effective safeguarding policies and procedures.;

Children's Trusts. The Act encourages the establishment of Children's Trusts, which bring together local authorities, health services, education providers, and other agencies to work collaboratively to improve outcomes for children and families. Children's Trusts are tasked with developing and implementing integrated services that meet the needs of children and young people in their area;

Information Sharing. The Children Act 2004 promotes the sharing of information between relevant agencies to support early intervention and safeguarding efforts. It reinforces the importance of effective communication and collaboration between professionals working with children and families to identify and respond to concerns at the earliest opportunity.

Common Assessment Framework (CAF). The Act introduces the Common Assessment Framework (CAF), a standardised tool for assessing the needs of children and identifying appropriate support services. The CAF aims to ensure that children and families receive coordinated support tailored to their individual needs, promoting better outcomes and reducing the risk of harm.

Many of these amendments and enhancements to child welfare legislation were instigated in the wake of the harrowing and, tragically, avoidable death of Victoria Climbié in 2000. The introduction of the Every Child Matters framework stemmed directly from the profound lessons gleaned from this heartbreaking case. Subsequent to the public inquest into Victoria's tragically short life and death, presided over by Lord Laming, a pivotal transformation in child welfare policy was set in motion. I will discuss the Victoria Climbié case further in this book as we look at individual case studies.

The legacy of the Children Act continues to shape child welfare policy and practice in the UK, hammering home the importance of collaboration, early intervention, and a child-centred approach in safeguarding and promoting the well-being of children and families.

<u>**Adults**</u>

The **Care Act 2014** singularly the most significant piece of legislation in the United Kingdom in terms of safeguarding adults at risk. It reformed the law relating to their care and support, as well as support for carers. The main provisions are this:

Adult Social Care - The Care Act introduces a range of reforms to adult social care in England. It aims to promote the well-being of individuals in need of care and support, the prevention and early intervention, as well as the integration of health and social care services;

Eligibility for Care and Support - The Act introduces a national eligibility threshold for care and support needs assessments. Local authorities must assess an individual's care and support needs, and if they meet the eligibility criteria, the local authority must arrange for the provision of necessary care and support;

Carers' Rights - The Care Act recognizes the vital role of unpaid carers and introduces new rights and support for them. Local authorities must assess carers' needs for support and provide services to meet those needs if eligible. Carers are entitled to the same assessment and support rights as the individuals they care for;

Safeguarding - The Act strengthens safeguarding adults at risk of abuse or neglect. Local authorities have a duty to make inquiries if they believe an adult is at risk and take action to protect them from harm;

Information and Advice - The Act requires local authorities to provide information and advice on care and support services available in their area. This includes signposting to relevant services and guidance on how to access support;

Scrutiny of Care Provision - The Care Act introduces measures to improve the quality and sustainability of care services by promoting transparency, accountability, and market stability. It includes provisions for monitoring the financial health of care providers and intervening where necessary to prevent service disruption;

Integration of Health and Social Care - The Act promotes greater integration between health and social care services to improve outcomes for individuals with care needs. This includes joint working arrangements between local authorities and the National Health Service (NHS) to coordinate care and support;

Deferred Payment Agreements - The Act enables individuals to enter into deferred payment agreements with their local authority to help cover the cost of residential care. This allows individuals to delay paying for their care until a later date, such as after their death or the sale of their home.

The Care Act 2014 in the United Kingdom is underpinned by six key principles that guide the provision of care and support services. These principles are:

The promotion of the person's wellbeing - The Care Act promotes the well-being of individuals with care and support needs and their carers. This includes considering their physical, mental, and emotional health, as well as their social and economic circumstances, and working to improve their overall quality of life;

Prevention - The Act stresses the importance of preventing or delaying the need for care and support through early intervention, prevention, and promoting independence. This involves identifying risks and providing support to address them before they escalate;

Empowering Individuals - The Care Act seeks to empower individuals to have control over their own care and support. It promotes choice and control, ensuring that individuals are involved in decisions about their care, and have the information and support they need to make informed choices;

Collaborating with Individuals - The Act promotes collaborative working between individuals, their families, carers, and care professionals. It recognizes the importance of involving individuals in decisions about their care and support, as well as consulting with them on the design and delivery of services;

Providing Information and Advice - The Care Act requires local authorities to provide information and advice to individuals and carers about care and support services available in their area. This includes signposting to relevant services, guidance on accessing support, and information about rights and entitlements;

Ensuring a Person-Centric Approach - The Act underlines the importance of providing care and support that is tailored to the individual needs and preferences of each person. This involves conducting person-centred assessments, developing care plans that reflect individual goals and preferences, and reviewing support arrangements regularly to ensure they remain appropriate and effective.

These principles are central to the ethos of the Care Act and provide the backbone for its aims of promoting well-being, preventing the need for care, empowering individuals, and ensuring that care and support services are delivered in a person-centred, collaborative, and holistic manner.

<u>Other legislation</u>

Safeguarding Vulnerable Groups Act 2006

The Safeguarding Vulnerable Groups Act 2006 (SVGA) is a piece of legislation in the United Kingdom aimed at protecting children and vulnerable adults from harm. It established the Disclosure and Barring Service (DBS) and created regulations surrounding the disclosure of information about individuals working with vulnerable groups. This act was introduced in response to growing concerns about the safety and protection of vulnerable individuals, particularly children and adults at risk, from abuse and harm.

Its primary purpose is to prevent unsuitable individuals from working with children and vulnerable adults, thereby safeguarding them from harm. One of the key provisions of the SVGA is the establishment of the Disclosure and Barring Service (DBS). This service merges the functions of the Criminal Records Bureau (CRB) and the Independent Safeguarding Authority (ISA). The DBS is responsible for processing requests for criminal records checks (DBS checks) for individuals working with vulnerable groups, including children and adults at risk.

The SVGA defines certain "regulated activities" that involve working with vulnerable groups. These activities include roles such as teaching, healthcare, social work, and roles in voluntary organisations. Individuals working in regulated activities are required to undergo DBS checks to ensure they are suitable to work with vulnerable groups. To ensure the effectiveness of this in the longer term, the SVGA establishes two barred lists. One for individuals barred from working with children and another for individuals barred from working with vulnerable adults. Employers and organisations are legally required to check these lists before hiring individuals for positions that involve working with vulnerable groups.

The SVGA places a duty on employers and certain professional bodies to make referrals to the DBS if they believe an individual poses a risk of harm to vulnerable groups. Failure to make a required referral can result in penalties, including criminal prosecution. The SVGA mandates continuous monitoring and review of individuals working with vulnerable groups. This includes ongoing criminal record checks and updates to barred lists as necessary. The SVGA aims to protect vulnerable groups, including children and adults at risk, from harm and abuse by ensuring that individuals working with them are suitable and safe to do so. It provides a framework for promoting safer recruitment practices and maintaining high standards of safeguarding across various sectors.

Since its enactment, the SVGA has been subject to amendments and updates to strengthen safeguarding measures and address emerging risks and challenges.

Working Together to Safeguard Children is statutory guidance issued by the UK government in 1999 that sets out the responsibilities of organisations and professionals in safeguarding and promoting the welfare of children. It provides a framework for inter-agency cooperation and collaboration to ensure that children are protected from abuse, neglect, and exploitation.

It is published by the Department for Education and provides statutory guidance under the Children Act 1989 and the Children and Social Work Act 2017. The guidance aims to ensure that all agencies and professionals involved in safeguarding children work together effectively to identify, assess, and respond to concerns about children's welfare.

The guidance is underpinned by key principles, including putting the needs and best interests of children first, taking a child-centred approach, and promoting early help and intervention to prevent harm. The guidance outlines the specific roles and responsibilities of different agencies and professionals involved in safeguarding, including local authorities, health services, schools, the police, and voluntary organisations. Most importantly for us, it clarifies the duties of designated safeguarding leads within organisations and the importance of multi-agency collaboration in safeguarding children.

The guidance goes on to set out the processes for identifying and responding to concerns about children's welfare, including procedures for making referrals to children's social care, conducting assessments, and developing child protection plans. It places great emphasis of robust risk assessment, information sharing, and joint working between agencies to ensure timely and appropriate interventions.

Working Together to Safeguard Children provides guidance on the conduct of child protection conferences and reviews, which are multi-agency meetings convened to assess the risks to a child and determine appropriate safeguarding measures.
It outlines the roles and responsibilities of professionals involved in conferences and reviews, as well as the process for reviewing and updating child protection plans.

This guidance includes provisions for conducting serious case reviews (SCRs) following cases where a child dies or is seriously harmed as a result of abuse or neglect. SCRs aim to identify lessons to be learned and improve safeguarding practice and puts a close focus on the importance of sharing learning from SCRs to inform policy, practice, and training at both local and national levels.

Working Together to Safeguard Children highlights the importance of training and professional development for individuals working with children and families, including DSLs, frontline practitioners, and managers. It recommends regular training on safeguarding policies, procedures, and best practice to ensure that professionals have the knowledge and skills to safeguard children effectively. The guidance promotes a culture of continuous improvement and accountability in safeguarding practice. It encourages agencies to monitor and evaluate their safeguarding arrangements, seek feedback from children and families, and take action to address any areas for improvement.

Recognising signs of abuse and neglect.

Recognising signs of abuse is a critical aspect of effective safeguarding efforts, enabling professionals and caregivers to identify potential risks and intervene promptly to protect those in need. This following section aims to provide a comprehensive overview of the signs and indicators of abuse across different forms of maltreatment, including physical, emotional, sexual, and neglect.

Understanding the signs of abuse requires a nuanced approach that considers individual circumstances, cultural factors, and the dynamics of relationships. This is a process that we refer to as 'contextualised safeguarding'. It is essential for practitioners, caregivers, and community members to be vigilant and proactive in recognizing signs of abuse, as early intervention can significantly mitigate harm and prevent further escalation of abuse.

Throughout this chapter, we will explore common signs and indicators associated with various forms of abuse, providing practical guidance on how to recognize and respond to concerns effectively. We will also discuss the importance of multi-agency collaboration, information sharing, and adherence to safeguarding policies and procedures in safeguarding efforts.

By equipping you with the knowledge and skills to recognize signs of abuse, we aim to empower individuals and organisations to fulfil their duty to safeguard vulnerable individuals and promote a culture of safety, respect, and protection for all. Together, we can make a meaningful difference in the lives of those at risk of abuse and neglect, ensuring that they receive the support and protection they need to thrive.

More about Contextualised Safeguarding.

Contextualised safeguarding is an approach to safeguarding vulnerable individuals, particularly children and young people, that recognizes the impact of broader environmental factors on their safety and well-being. It acknowledges that risks to individuals often arise from their social and physical environments, such as peer groups, families, schools, neighbourhoods, and digital/online spaces. Contextual safeguarding seeks to understand and address these risks within the specific contexts in which they occur, rather than focusing solely on individual behaviours or incidents of harm.

Key components of contextual safeguarding include:

Understanding Contexts - Contextual safeguarding recognizes that individuals' experiences of abuse and harm are influenced by the environments in which they live, learn, and socialise. This includes factors such as family dynamics, peer relationships, community norms, socio-economic conditions, and access to support services.

Assessing Multiple Risks - Instead of solely focusing on risks within the home environment, contextual safeguarding adopts a broader perspective, considering risks that may arise in various contexts, including schools, neighbourhoods, online spaces, and peer groups. This involves assessing the influence of social networks, community dynamics, and wider systemic factors on individuals' safety and well-being.

Intervening Across Systems - Contextual safeguarding recognizes that addressing risks to individuals often requires interventions across multiple systems and sectors, including social services, education, health, law enforcement, and community organisations. It emphasises the importance of collaboration and partnership working to coordinate responses and support individuals effectively.

Empowering Communities - Contextual safeguarding involves engaging with communities and stakeholders to understand local contexts, identify strengths and resources, and develop tailored interventions that address underlying risks and promote protective factors. This may include initiatives to strengthen community networks, increase access to support services, and empower individuals to recognize and respond to risks within their communities.

Adapting Practice - Practitioners working within a contextual safeguarding framework are encouraged to adapt their practice to better address environmental risks and support individuals in diverse contexts. This may involve developing specialised skills in areas such as risk assessment, multi-agency working, and trauma-informed practice, as well as promoting cultural competence and sensitivity to individuals' diverse backgrounds and experiences.

Contextualised safeguarding represents a shift towards a more holistic and inclusive approach to safeguarding vulnerable individuals, recognising the interconnectedness of social, environmental, and individual factors in shaping experiences of abuse and harm. By addressing risks within their broader contexts, contextualised safeguarding seeks to create safer and more supportive environments for all individuals, enabling them to thrive and reach their full potential.

<u>**Physical Abuse**</u>

Physical abuse refers to the intentional use of force or violence against another person that results in physical harm, injury, pain, or impairment. It is a form of abuse that can occur in various settings, including within families, intimate relationships, institutions, schools, workplaces, and communities. Physical abuse can take many forms, ranging from hitting, punching, kicking, and slapping to more severe acts such as burning, scalding, choking, or using weapons against the victim.

Physical abuse is a criminal offence and also a violation of human rights. Victims of physical abuse may require medical attention, counselling, and support services to address the physical and emotional effects of the abuse, particularly when the abuse is perpetrated during childhood.

Physical indicators of physical abuse include:

• Unexplained bruises, welts, or marks on the body, particularly in areas not commonly injured accidentally (e.g., back, buttocks, thighs).

• Bruises or injuries in varied stages of healing.

• Patterned or shaped bruises (e.g., belt buckle marks, hand/palm prints).

• Multiple or repeated injuries, especially with inconsistent or vague explanations.

• Burns or scalds, including cigarette burns, immersion burns, or burns in unusual shapes or patterns.

• Fractures, particularly in non-weight-bearing bones such as ribs or the skull.

• Head injuries, including signs of skull fractures or traumatic brain injuries.

• Facial injuries, such as black eyes, swollen lips, or broken teeth.

• Bite marks or other evidence of human or animal bites

• Lacerations, abrasions, or cuts, especially those with irregular or linear patterns.

• Internal injuries, evidenced by abdominal pain, vomiting blood, or blood in the stool.

• Swelling or tenderness in various body parts.

- Signs of strangulation, such as petechiae (tiny red spots) around the neck.

- Genital or anal injuries, including bruising, bleeding, or tears.

- Signs of malnutrition or dehydration, such as sunken eyes, pale skin, or poor growth.
- Failure to thrive or significant weight loss without medical explanation.

- Overuse of medication or inappropriate administration of medication.

- Signs of neglect, such as poor hygiene, untreated medical conditions, or inadequate clothing.

- Wearing loose covering clothing, even during hot weather.

- Self-harming behaviors or suicide attempts, especially in older children and adolescents.

Emotional indicators of physical abuse include:

- **Fearfulness** - Victims may exhibit heightened fearfulness, particularly in the presence of certain individuals or in specific situations.

- **Anxiety** - Victims may display symptoms of anxiety, including restlessness, irritability, nervousness, or excessive worrying.

- **Withdrawal** - Victims may withdraw from social interactions or activities they previously enjoyed. They may become quiet, introverted, or avoidant of others.

- **Depression** - Victims may exhibit symptoms of depression, such as persistent sadness, tearfulness, hopelessness, or loss of interest in activities.

- **Low Self-Esteem** - Victims may have low self-esteem and feelings of worthlessness. They may express negative self-talk or exhibit self-deprecating behaviour.

- **Aggression** - Victims may display aggressive behaviours, such as outbursts of anger, hostility, or aggression towards others or objects.

- **Emotional Instability** - Victims may experience emotional volatility, with sudden mood swings or intense emotional reactions disproportionate to the situation.

- **Regression** - Victims may exhibit regressive behaviours, reverting to earlier developmental stages, such as bedwetting, thumb-sucking, or clinging to caregivers.

- **Avoidance:** Victims may avoid certain individuals, places, or activities associated with the abuse. They may express reluctance to go home or be alone with specific caregivers.

- **Guilt or Shame** - Victims may experience feelings of guilt or shame, blaming themselves for the abuse or feeling embarrassed about their experiences.

- **Sleep Disturbances** - Victims may experience disruptions in sleep patterns, including difficulty falling asleep, nightmares, or night terrors.

- **Social Isolation** - Victims may become socially isolated, having difficulty forming and maintaining friendships or participating in social activities.

- **Academic Decline** - Children's academic performance may decline, with difficulties concentrating, completing tasks, or retaining information.

- **Risk-Taking Behaviors** - Victims may engage in risky or self-destructive behaviors, such as substance abuse, self-harm, or suicidal ideation.

- **Substance Abuse** - Adults may turn to alcohol or drugs as a way to cope with emotional pain or numb their feelings.

- **Suicidal Thoughts** - Adults may experience thoughts of suicide or self-harm as a result of the emotional pain and despair caused by the abuse.

As safeguarders we must learn and appreciate that emotional signs of physical abuse can vary widely among individuals and may not always be immediately apparent. Additionally, individuals may exhibit a combination of these signs or symptoms, and they may fluctuate over time.

There are several ways we can support **adult** victims of physical abuse:

Listen and Believe - Provide a safe and non-judgmental space for the victim to share their experiences. Validate their feelings and experiences by actively listening and believing their account of the abuse.

Offer Emotional Support - Offer empathy, compassion, and emotional support to the victim. Let them know that they are not alone and that you are there to support them through their journey of healing.

Respect Their Choices - Respect the victim's autonomy and empower them to make their own decisions. Avoid pressuring them into taking actions they are not comfortable with and support them in whatever choices they make regarding their safety and well-being.

Provide Practical Assistance - Offer practical assistance such as helping them find resources and support services in their community, accompanying them to appointments or meetings, or assisting with tasks they may find challenging due to the abuse.

Encourage Professional Help - Encourage the victim to seek professional help from trained professionals such as counsellors, therapists, or support groups. Provide information about available resources and services that may be helpful for them.

Safety Planning - Help the victim create a safety plan to protect themselves from further harm. This may involve identifying safe places to go in case of emergency, setting boundaries with the abuser, and developing strategies to stay safe.

Educate Yourself - Educate yourself about the dynamics of physical abuse, signs of abuse, and available resources for victims. This will enable you to provide more effective support and assistance to the victim.

Be Patient and Persistent - Be patient and understanding with the victim, as healing from physical abuse can be a long and difficult process. Offer your support consistently and persistently, even if the victim is not ready to accept help immediately.

Supporting **children** who have been or are suspect of being physically abused is somewhat more nuanced.

Report Suspected Abuse - If you suspect a child is being physically abused, report your concerns to the appropriate authorities, such as child protective services or law enforcement. Reporting suspected abuse is crucial in ensuring the safety and well-being of the child.

Listen and Believe - Provide a safe and supportive environment for the child to share their experiences. Listen to them without judgement and believe their account of the abuse. Let them know that it is not their fault and that they are not alone.

Offer Emotional Support - Offer comfort, empathy, and reassurance to the child. Let them know that you care about them and are there to support them through this difficult time. Encourage them to express their feelings and emotions in a safe and healthy way.

Encourage Disclosure - Encourage the child to talk about their experiences and feelings, but do not pressure them to disclose if they are not ready. Let them know that it is okay to talk about what happened and that you are there to listen and help.

Be Patient and Understanding - Be patient and understanding with the child as they process their experiences and emotions. Healing from physical abuse takes time, and the child may need support and reassurance along the way.

Connect Them with Support Services - Connect the child with support services such as counseling, therapy, or support groups for child abuse survivors. These services can provide the child with the help and resources they need to heal and recover from the abuse.

Educate Yourself - Educate yourself about the signs of physical abuse, the impact it can have on children, and how to provide effective support. This will enable you to better understand the child's needs and offer more effective assistance.

<u>**Sexual Abuse**</u>

Conversations concerning sexual abuse, especially when it pertains to the abuse of children, can and does evoke strong emotional responses. This subject matter is profoundly sensitive, often capable of triggering trauma reactions in survivors and deep-seated anger in those who have not experienced such abuse firsthand.

Sexual abuse is any mistreatment of another person characterised by non-consensual sexual acts or behavior imposed on an individual without their consent or understanding. It encompasses a wide range of actions, including but not limited to sexual assault / inappropriate touching, rape, molestation, coercion, exploitation, and harassment. Sexual abuse can occur within various contexts, including familial relationships (incest), intimate partnerships, institutional and educational settings, or by individuals in positions of authority or trust. It inflicts profound physical, psychological, and emotional harm on victims, often causing lasting trauma, shame, and interpersonal difficulties.

Physical indicators of sexual abuse include:

- Unexplained injuries to the genital or anal area, such as bruising, bleeding, or tearing.

- Difficulty walking or sitting, particularly if there is pain or discomfort in the genital or anal region.

- Sexually transmitted infections (STIs) or other genital infections.

- Pregnancy in a child or adolescent.

- Signs of trauma or injury to other parts of the body, such as bruises, scratches, or bite marks.

- Changes in behaviour, mood, or personality, such as withdrawal, aggression, or depression.

- Sleep disturbances, nightmares, or bedwetting.

- Regression in behaviour, such as reverting to bedwetting or thumb sucking.

- Fear or anxiety related to specific people, places, or activities.

- Self-harming behaviors or suicide attempts.

- Sudden changes in appetite or weight loss.

- Excessive grooming or hygiene rituals, such as frequent bathing or washing the genital area.
- Inappropriate sexual knowledge, language, or behaviour for the child's age. This includes overtly displayed sexualised language that appears to beyond the years of the suspected survivor.

- Avoidance of physical contact or discomfort with affectionate gestures.

- Sexualized play or drawings that are inappropriate for the child's age.

Identifying emotional symptoms of sexual abuse in both adults and children can prove challenging, as they often overlap with manifestations of other forms of abuse or neglect. Nonetheless, the following signs may be observed:

- **Fear and Anxiety**: Children or adults who have experienced sexual abuse may exhibit fear or anxiety, particularly in situations or around individuals that remind them of the abuse. They may have irrational fears or experience panic attacks.

- **Depression:** Feelings of sadness, hopelessness, and despair are common emotional responses to sexual abuse. Children or adults may lose interest in activities they once enjoyed and may struggle with feelings of worthlessness or guilt.

- **Withdrawal:** Children or adults may withdraw from social interactions, preferring to be alone rather than spending time with friends or family members. They may become increasingly isolated and may have difficulty trusting others.
- **Aggression:** Some Children or adults may display aggressive behaviour as a way of expressing their anger and frustration. They may lash out at others verbally or physically, or exhibit impulsive and reckless behaviour.

- **Low Self-Esteem:** Sexual abuse can shatter a child or adult's sense of self-worth and lead to feelings of inadequacy or self-doubt. Children or adults may struggle with low self-esteem and may engage in self-destructive behaviours as a result.
- **Mood Swings:** Children or adults who have experienced sexual abuse may exhibit sudden and unpredictable changes in mood. They may seem fine one moment and then become irritable, angry, or tearful without apparent cause.

- **Guilt and Shame:** Children or adults often experience feelings of guilt and shame following sexual abuse, even though they are not at fault. They may blame themselves for the abuse or feel ashamed of what happened, leading to a reluctance to disclose the abuse or seek help.

- **Sleep Disturbances:** Nightmares, insomnia, and other sleep disturbances are common emotional responses to sexual abuse. Children or adults may have difficulty falling asleep or staying asleep and may experience recurring nightmares related to the abuse.

- **Difficulty Concentrating:** Sexual abuse can interfere with a child or adult's ability to concentrate and focus on tasks. They may struggle academically or have difficulty completing assignments or following instructions.
- **Self-Harming Behaviors:** Some Children or adults may engage in self-harming behaviors as a way of coping with the emotional pain and trauma of sexual abuse. This can include cutting, burning, or other forms of self-injury.

As safeguarders, we regard disclosures of sexual abuse as a huge priority for several critical reasons. The primary concern is the immediate safety and well-being of the victim. Sexual abuse can cause significant physical, emotional, and psychological harm, and it's crucial to intervene promptly to prevent further abuse and mitigate the impact of trauma on the victim.

Disclosures of sexual abuse provide an opportunity to prevent further victimization. By taking swift and decisive action in response to disclosures, we can remove the victim from harm's way, prevent the perpetrator from inflicting additional abuse, and safeguard other potential victims from similar harm. Prompt intervention following a disclosure of sexual abuse is essential for facilitating the victim's healing and recovery process. Providing victims with access to appropriate support services, such as counselling, therapy, medical care, and advocacy, can help them cope with the aftermath of the abuse, address trauma-related symptoms, and rebuild their lives.

By responding effectively to disclosures of sexual abuse, we can implement preventative measures to address systemic issues, improve safeguarding practices, and create safer environments for children and vulnerable individuals. This may involve implementing policies and procedures to prevent future abuse, providing training and education on recognizing and responding to abuse, and promoting awareness and advocacy efforts to challenge cultural norms and attitudes that enable abuse to occur.

Prioritizing disclosures of sexual abuse is essential for ensuring the safety, well-being, and rights of victims and creating a culture of safety, transparency, and accountability within our communities. By responding with urgency, compassion, and expertise to disclosures of sexual abuse, we can make meaningful strides toward preventing abuse and supporting survivors.

Safeguarders have a vital role in supporting child victims of sexual abuse. First and foremost, it's crucial to create a safe and supportive environment for the child to share their experiences. Listen to them with empathy and without judgement, allowing them to express their feelings and concerns. Believe their account of the abuse and reassure them that they are not alone. Encourage the child to seek help from trusted adults, such as parents, teachers, or counsellors, and offer to accompany them if they feel scared or unsure. Provide emotional support by offering comfort, validation, and reassurance throughout their healing journey. Educate yourself about the signs of sexual abuse and available resources for victims, enabling you to provide informed support and assistance. Finally, advocate for the child's safety and well-being by reporting suspected abuse to the appropriate authorities and supporting them in accessing the help they need to heal and recover.

<u>**Neglect**</u>

To comprehensively grasp the concept of neglect, it is essential to delineate and examine its three distinct subtypes.

Neglect refers to the failure to provide necessary care, support, or resources to meet an individual's basic needs, resulting in harm or impairment to their physical, emotional, or psychological well-being. Neglect can occur in various contexts, including within families, institutions, or caregiving relationships. Examples of neglect may include failure to provide adequate food, shelter, clothing, medical care, supervision, or emotional support. Neglect can have severe and long-lasting consequences, particularly for vulnerable populations such as children, elderly individuals, or individuals with disabilities.

Self-Neglect occurs when an individual fails to adequately care for themselves, leading to harm or endangerment of their own health, safety, or well-being. Self-neglect can manifest in various ways, including neglecting personal hygiene, nutrition, medical care, or living conditions. Common indicators of self-neglect may include unkempt appearance, malnutrition, hoarding, refusal of necessary medical treatment, or living in unsafe or unsanitary conditions. Self-neglect can be particularly concerning among elderly individuals or individuals with physical or mental health challenges who may struggle to meet their own needs.

Wilful Neglect refers to neglect that occurs intentionally or knowingly, with the perpetrator deliberately failing to provide necessary care or support despite being capable of doing so. Unlike unintentional or passive neglect, which may result from factors such as lack of awareness, resources, or ability, wilful neglect involves a conscious decision to withhold care or assistance. Wilful neglect may involve malicious intent, indifference, or disregard for the well-being of the individual affected. It is often considered a serious form of abuse or mistreatment and may result in legal consequences for the perpetrator. Examples of wilful neglect may include intentionally withholding food or medication, denying access to medical care, or abandoning a dependent individual in unsafe conditions.

In the UK Wilful neglect is a criminal offence. The penalties vary depending on the severity of the offence and the context in which it occurs. However, wilful neglect is considered a serious offence, particularly in cases involving vulnerable individuals such as children, elderly persons, or individuals with disabilities. Penalties for wilful neglect may include fines, imprisonment, or both.

For healthcare professionals, including doctors, nurses, and caregivers, wilful neglect can result in professional disciplinary action, including suspension or revocation of a professional licence or registration (being struck-off). Additionally, individuals found guilty of wilful neglect may be subject to civil liability, including compensation claims for damages suffered by the victim as a result of the neglect. In cases involving institutional neglect, such as neglect occurring in care homes, hospitals, or educational institutions, the responsible institution may face legal sanctions, including fines, closure orders, or regulatory enforcement action.

The specific legal penalties for wilful neglect are outlined in various laws and regulations, including the Criminal Law Act 1977, the Mental Capacity Act 2005, the Care Act 2014, and the Health and Social Care Act 2008 (Regulated Activities) Regulations 2014, among others.

The term **acts of omission** refers to instances where an individual or entity fails to take necessary action or fulfil a duty, resulting in harm or detriment to another person. This can include neglecting to provide essential care, support, or resources, as well as failing to intervene in situations where intervention is required to prevent harm. Acts of omission can occur in various contexts, such as caregiving, parenting, professional responsibilities, or legal obligations. Neglect, on the other hand, is a specific type of act of omission that involves the failure to provide necessary care, support, or resources to meet an individual's basic needs, resulting in harm or impairment to their physical, emotional, or psychological well-being. While all acts of neglect are acts of omission, not all acts of omission constitute neglect. Neglect typically involves a pattern of ongoing failure to meet a person's needs, whereas acts of omission may occur as isolated incidents or as part of a broader pattern of behaviour.

The warning signs of neglect in adults can vary depending on the specific circumstances and the type of neglect involved. However, some common warning signs of neglect in adults include:

Poor Hygiene - Neglected adults may exhibit signs of poor personal hygiene, such as unwashed clothes, body odour, unkempt hair, or untreated medical conditions.

Malnutrition or Dehydration - Adults who are neglected may show signs of malnutrition or dehydration, including significant weight loss, sunken eyes, dry skin, or frequent illnesses related to poor nutrition.

Untreated Medical Conditions - Neglected adults may have untreated medical conditions or injuries that are left unattended due to a lack of access to healthcare or neglectful caregiving.

Unsafe Living Conditions - Neglected adults may live in unsafe or unsanitary conditions, such as cluttered or dirty living spaces, inadequate heating or cooling, or exposure to hazards such as mould, pests, or fire risks.

Social Isolation - Neglected adults may exhibit signs of social isolation or withdrawal from social activities, family, or friends. They may lack meaningful social connections and may have limited contact with others.

Financial Exploitation - Neglected adults may be vulnerable to financial exploitation, such as unpaid bills, overdue rent or mortgage payments, or unauthorised use of their finances by others.

Emotional Distress - Neglected adults may experience emotional distress or psychological symptoms related to their neglect, such as depression, anxiety, low self-esteem, or feelings of worthlessness.

Lack of Basic Necessities - Neglected adults may lack access to basic necessities such as food, water, clothing, shelter, or medication. They may struggle to meet their daily needs due to neglectful caregiving or inadequate resources.

Unmet Personal Care Needs - Neglected adults may have unmet personal care needs, such as assistance with bathing, toileting, dressing, or mobility. They may be unable to perform daily tasks independently due to neglect.

Decline in Functioning - Neglected adults may experience a decline in their physical or cognitive functioning as a result of neglect, leading to difficulties in performing daily activities or maintaining independence.

Many of these might also be red flags for neglect in children. Additionally we may see:

- Persistent hunger, malnutrition, or signs of undernourishment, such as being significantly underweight or having a distended abdomen.
- Poor hygiene, including unwashed clothes, body odour, or untreated dental issues.
- Inadequate clothing for the weather conditions, such as being poorly dressed in cold weather.
- Untreated medical conditions or injuries, such as infections, untreated illnesses, or injuries left unattended.
- Failure to thrive, with developmental delays or growth retardation compared to peers.
- Chronic absenteeism from school or frequent tardiness.
- Lack of appropriate school supplies or inadequate participation in educational activities.
- Difficulty concentrating, learning, or completing homework assignments due to hunger, fatigue, or emotional distress.
- Withdrawal or social isolation from peers and adults.
- Persistent sadness, depression, or anxiety.

- Low self-esteem, feelings of worthlessness, or self-blame.
- Aggressive or disruptive behaviour, possibly as a way to attract attention or cope with feelings of neglect.
- Difficulty forming attachments or trusting others.
- Avoidance of eye contact or physical contact with caregivers.
- Lack of appropriate supervision, such as being left alone for extended periods or being cared for by inadequately trained or irresponsible caregivers.
- Engaging in risky behaviours due to lack of supervision or guidance.
- Frequent accidents or injuries that could have been prevented with proper supervision or safety measures.
- Inconsistent access to food, leading to hoarding or stealing food.
- Inadequate clothing or footwear for weather conditions.
- Insecure or unstable housing situations, such as frequent moves or living in unsafe or overcrowded conditions.
- Parental substance abuse or mental health issues that impair their ability to provide adequate care and supervision.
- Neglectful or indifferent parenting behaviours, such as ignoring the child's needs, minimising their concerns, or failing to seek help when needed.
- Educational and Developmental Delays
- Significant delays in reaching developmental milestones, such as walking, talking, or potty training.
- Poor academic performance or delays in cognitive development due to lack of stimulation, support, or consistent caregiving.

By recognizing the signs and indicators of neglect, implementing robust prevention strategies, and intervening promptly when concerns arise, safeguarding professionals can play a crucial role in protecting individuals from harm and promoting their safety, dignity, and rights.

In our role we always play our part in supporting victims of neglect through various means. Firstly, it's essential to recognize the signs of neglect as listed above so that we may identify individuals who may be experiencing neglect and offer our assistance. Secondly, we can provide practical support by offering resources and connecting them with relevant services, such as food banks, shelters, healthcare providers, or social services agencies. Additionally, offering emotional support and a listening ear can be invaluable to someone experiencing neglect, providing them with a sense of validation and understanding. By advocating for their needs and rights, we can help ensure that victims of neglect receive the support and assistance they require to address their situation and improve their well-being.

Through making a referral, we ensure that our concerns regarding suspected neglect are diligently investigated and appropriately addressed. By directing our concerns to the local authority children's service team who are equipped to intervene, we initiate a process whereby the circumstances prompting our suspicions are thoroughly scrutinised. This will enable timely and necessary actions to be taken, ensuring the welfare and safety of those potentially affected by neglect.

<u>**Psychological abuse.**</u>

Psychological abuse, also known as emotional abuse, encompasses a range of behaviours and tactics aimed at undermining an individual's sense of self-worth, autonomy, and well-being. This form of abuse involves the use of verbal, non-verbal, or covert actions to control, manipulate, intimidate, or belittle the victim, causing profound emotional and psychological harm. Examples of psychological abuse may include verbal insults, threats, gaslighting, humiliation, isolation, and manipulation. Unlike physical abuse, psychological abuse often leaves no visible scars, making it challenging to detect and address. However, its impact can be equally devastating, resulting in long-lasting emotional trauma, low self-esteem, anxiety, depression, and difficulty forming healthy relationships. Recognising the signs of psychological abuse and providing support and intervention are crucial in protecting individuals from its harmful effects and promoting their emotional well-being.

Signs that an adult might be a victim of psychological abuse can vary, but some common indicators include:

Low Self-Esteem - Individuals experiencing psychological abuse may exhibit low self-esteem and a lack of confidence in themselves. They may express feelings of worthlessness or self-doubt.

Anxiety and Depression - Victims of psychological abuse often experience anxiety, depression, or other mental health issues as a result of the constant emotional manipulation and control exerted by the abuser.

Social Withdrawal - Victims may withdraw from social interactions and isolate themselves from friends, family, and support networks. They may become increasingly isolated as the abuser seeks to control their access to others.

Changes in Behaviour - Victims of psychological abuse may exhibit changes in behaviour, such as becoming more passive, submissive, or fearful. They may also display signs of agitation, irritability, or mood swings.

Constant Criticism - Psychological abusers frequently criticise and belittle their victims, often in front of others. Victims may internalise this criticism and believe that they are incompetent or unworthy.

Fear of the Abuser - Victims of psychological abuse may live in constant fear of their abuser and may go to great lengths to avoid confrontation or conflict. They may also exhibit physical symptoms of stress or trauma in the abuser's presence.

Loss of Independence - Psychological abusers often seek to control every aspect of their victim's life, leading to a loss of independence and autonomy. Victims may feel unable to make decisions or take action without the abuser's approval.

Self-Blame - Victims of psychological abuse may internalise the blame for the abuse, believing that they somehow deserve the mistreatment or that they are responsible for changing the abuser's behaviour.

Physical Symptoms - Psychological abuse can have physical manifestations, such as headaches, digestive issues, insomnia, or other stress-related ailments.

In children, additional signs of psychological abuse may include:

Regression - Children may exhibit regressive behaviours such as bedwetting, thumb sucking, or clinginess, particularly if they were previously toilet trained or independent.

Fearfulness - Children may display excessive fear or anxiety, particularly around specific individuals or situations. They may also express fear of making mistakes or displeasing others.

Avoidance - Children may avoid certain activities, places, or people associated with the abuser or situations where they have experienced psychological abuse.

Emotional Instability - Children may have difficulty regulating their emotions and may display frequent mood swings, outbursts of anger or sadness, or emotional numbing.

Social Withdrawal - Children may withdraw from social interactions with peers, family members, or trusted adults. They may become increasingly isolated and have difficulty forming or maintaining friendships.

Changes in Behavior at School - Children may exhibit changes in behaviour or academic performance at school, such as a decline in grades, disruptive behaviour, or difficulty concentrating.

Excessive Apologising - Children may apologise excessively or blame themselves for situations beyond their control, as they may have been conditioned to believe they are responsible for the abuse.

Developmental Delays - Psychological abuse can impact a child's cognitive, social, and emotional development, leading to delays in reaching developmental milestones.

Psychosomatic Symptoms - Children may experience physical symptoms such as headaches, stomachaches, or fatigue that have no apparent medical cause but are related to stress or emotional distress.

Self-Harming Behaviours - In severe cases of psychological abuse, children may engage in self-harming behaviours such as cutting, scratching, or hitting themselves as a way to cope with emotional pain or express feelings of powerlessness.

Children may not always recognize or be able to articulate that they are experiencing psychological abuse. Additionally, signs of psychological abuse in children may overlap with other forms of abuse or trauma. If you suspect that a child is experiencing psychological abuse, it's crucial to take their concerns seriously, provide a supportive and validating environment, and seek help from appropriate professionals, such as child protective services or mental health professionals, to ensure the child's safety and well-being.

Supporting adult and child victims of emotional abuse requires a multifaceted approach that addresses their emotional, psychological, and practical needs. Firstly, it's crucial to provide a safe and supportive environment where victims feel comfortable expressing their feelings and concerns without fear of judgement. Actively listening to their experiences with empathy and validation can help them feel heard and understood. Encourage them to seek professional help from counsellors, therapists, or support groups specialising in emotional abuse, as these resources can provide invaluable guidance and support. Additionally, offering practical assistance, such as helping them access resources for housing, legal aid, or financial assistance, can help alleviate some of the burdens they may be facing. Finally, advocating for their rights and well-being by speaking out against emotional abuse and promoting awareness within the community can help reduce stigma and provide a supportive network for victims to turn to for help. By offering empathy, support, and practical assistance, we can help adult and child victims of emotional abuse navigate their healing journey and rebuild their sense of self-worth and empowerment.

<u>**Domestic Abuse**</u>

Domestic abuse describes a recurring pattern of behaviours deployed by one partner to assert and sustain dominance over the other within the context of an intimate relationship. Such behaviour transcends marital status or living arrangements, occurring in relationships encompassing marriage, cohabitation, dating, or any other form of intimate liaison, irrespective of the individuals' gender, sexual orientation, racial background, or socioeconomic standing.

This form of abusive behaviour encompasses a spectrum of injurious actions, comprising not only physical violence but also emotional and psychological abuse, sexual coercion, financial exploitation, and various forms of controlling conduct. While physical violence is a conspicuous manifestation, it is imperative to recognize that domestic abuse extends beyond overt acts of aggression. Verbal threats, intimidation tactics, social isolation, persistent surveillance, coercive tactics, and manipulative behaviours are equally prevalent components.

Additionally, the insidious nature of domestic abuse often results in its escalation over time, exacerbating its detrimental impact. Victims frequently endure enduring physical and psychological trauma, and the repercussions extend beyond the individual to affect children and other family members who may bear witness to or directly experience the abuse. Notably, with the enactment of the Domestic Abuse Act 2021, the classification of children who witness domestic abuse as victims, regardless of whether they are direct targets, underscores the recognition of the profound and pervasive impact of such trauma.

Coercive Control

Coercive control is an additional form of control that occurs within the home and in the context of domestic abuse. Unlike isolated incidents of physical violence, coercive control operates through a range of tactics aimed at instilling fear, dependency, and submission in the victim. It involves systematic efforts to undermine the victim's autonomy, self-esteem, and freedom, thereby trapping them in a cycle of abuse.

In the context of domestic abuse, coercive control manifests through various means, including:

Isolation - The abuser may isolate the victim from friends, family, and support networks, limiting their social interactions and cutting off avenues for seeking help or support.

Monitoring and Surveillance - This involves constant monitoring of the victim's activities, such as checking their phone, emails, or social media accounts, tracking their whereabouts, or using surveillance technology to keep tabs on them.

Manipulation and Gaslighting - Coercive control often entails psychological manipulation and gaslighting, where the abuser distorts reality, undermines the victim's perceptions, and makes them doubt their own thoughts, feelings, and experiences. The term "gaslighting" comes from the 1938 play "Gas Light" by Patrick Hamilton, later adapted into a 1944 film. In the story, a manipulative husband dims the gaslights to make his wife doubt her sanity.

Threats and Intimidation - The abuser may use threats of violence, harm, or retaliation to keep the victim compliant and submissive. This can include explicit threats as well as implied ones, creating an atmosphere of fear and apprehension.

Economic Abuse - Coercive control may also involve controlling the victim's finances, such as withholding money, preventing them from working or accessing financial resources, or sabotaging their attempts to become financially independent.

Emotional Abuse - This includes demeaning, belittling, or humiliating the victim, manipulating their emotions, and using guilt or shame to maintain control over them.

As coercive control persists, it incrementally chips away at the victim's self-esteem, autonomy, and capacity to act independently. This erosion often occurs insidiously, with the victim potentially oblivious to the gradual manipulation and domination unfolding within the relationship. The cumulative impact of coercive control extends far beyond the immediate circumstances, exerting profound and enduring consequences on both the victim's physical and psychological well-being.

The subtle nature of coercive control renders the victim vulnerable to a myriad of adverse effects, encompassing a broad spectrum of physical and mental health repercussions. Physically, the stress and anxiety induced by the sustained manipulation and intimidation can manifest in various somatic symptoms, ranging from chronic headaches and gastrointestinal issues to cardiovascular complications. Moreover, the pervasive emotional turmoil inflicted by coercive control can precipitate debilitating conditions such as depression, anxiety disorders, and post-traumatic stress disorder (PTSD).

Yet, perhaps equally formidable are the barriers that coercive control erects, impeding the victim's ability to extricate themselves from the abusive dynamic or seek assistance. The relentless erosion of self-worth and agency sows seeds of doubt and powerlessness, fostering a sense of dependency on the abuser and undermining the victim's belief in their capacity to effect change. Consequently, leaving the abusive relationship or reaching out for support becomes a daunting prospect, fraught with uncertainty, fear, and perceived risks.

In essence, the deceptive progression of coercive control poses formidable challenges for victims, enveloping them in a web of manipulation and intimidation that exacts a heavy toll on their physical, mental, and emotional well-being. Recognizing the complexities of coercive control is imperative for fostering empathy, understanding, and effective intervention strategies to support survivors and dismantle the pervasive cycle of abuse.

Supporting a victim of domestic abuse.

The principal steps taken by a safeguarding lead to provide assistance to a victim of domestic abuse would involve initiating a DASH (Domestic Abuse, Stalking, and Harassment) referral in collaboration with the police service. A professional working in social services or a similar field, would design a safety plan tailored to the specific needs and circumstances of the victim of domestic abuse. Here's a general outline of how they might approach creating such a plan:

Assessment - The safeguarding lead would conduct a thorough assessment of the victim's situation, taking into account factors such as the severity of the abuse, the presence of children or other dependents, the victim's access to resources, and any existing support networks.

Safety Planning Meeting - The safeguarding lead would meet with the victim in a safe and confidential environment to discuss their concerns, assess their immediate safety needs, and collaboratively develop a safety plan.

Identifying Risks -Together with the victim, the safeguarding lead would identify potential risks and danger points, such as times when the abuse is more likely to occur, triggers for the abuser's behaviour, and any potential barriers to leaving the abusive relationship.

Establishing Safety Measures - Based on the identified risks, the safeguarding lead would help the victim establish practical safety measures to minimise the risk of harm. This might include things like creating a code word or signal to alert others when they are in danger, identifying safe places to go in an emergency, and securing important documents and belongings.

Emergency Contact Information - The safeguarding lead would provide the victim with important emergency contact information, such as hotlines, shelters, and local law enforcement agencies, and help them develop a plan for how to access help quickly if needed.

Building Support Networks - The safeguarding lead would assist the victim in building and strengthening their support network, connecting them with community resources, support groups, counselling services, and other forms of assistance.

Self-Care Strategies - The safeguarding lead would help the victim develop self-care strategies to cope with the emotional and psychological effects of abuse, such as mindfulness techniques, relaxation exercises, and journaling.

Regular Review and Update - The safeguarding lead would periodically review and update the safety plan in response to changes in the victim's circumstances or the level of risk they are facing, ensuring that it remains effective and relevant over time.

Throughout the process, the safeguarding lead would prioritise the victim's safety, autonomy, and well-being, empowering them to make informed decisions and take action to protect themselves from further harm.

<u>**Financial Abuse**</u>

Financial abuse is any form of exploitation where an individual's financial resources or assets are improperly or illegally used by another person for personal gain or control. This type of abuse can occur in various relationships, including between partners, family members, caregivers, or trusted professionals. Financial abuse can take many forms, ranging from theft and fraud to coercion, manipulation, or undue influence over financial decisions. Examples include stealing money or property, forging signatures on financial documents, coercing someone into signing over control of their finances, or exploiting vulnerable individuals for financial gain.

Financial abuse can have significant and far-reaching consequences, including financial hardship, loss of assets, compromised financial security, and diminished independence and autonomy. Victims of financial abuse may experience feelings of powerlessness, shame, and betrayal, as well as difficulties in seeking help due to financial dependence on the abuser. It's essential to recognize the signs of financial abuse, including sudden changes in financial status, unexplained withdrawals or transfers, and discrepancies in financial records. Taking steps to prevent financial abuse, such as setting up safeguards, establishing power of attorney documents, and educating individuals about their financial rights and resources, can help protect against exploitation and promote financial security and well-being. Additionally, providing support and resources for survivors of financial abuse is crucial in helping them regain control over their finances and rebuild their lives.

Financial abuse manifests in various forms, each posing significant risks to individuals who are especially susceptible to exploitation or mistreatment. These distinct types of financial abuse can inflict profound harm on vulnerable individuals, compromising their financial security, autonomy, and overall well-being. It is imperative to recognize and understand these different types of financial abuse to effectively safeguard those who may be at risk and to implement preventative measures to mitigate the impact of such exploitation.

Theft - This involves the unauthorised taking or use of another person's money, property, or assets for personal gain.

Fraud - Fraudulent activities involve deception or misrepresentation to obtain money, assets, or financial information unlawfully. Examples include identity theft, credit card fraud, or investment scams.

Coercion - Coercion occurs when an individual uses threats, intimidation, or manipulation to control another person's financial decisions or resources.

Undue Influence - Undue influence involves exerting pressure or influence over someone to compel them to make financial decisions or transactions that benefit the influencer at the expense of the victim's best interests.

Exploitation - Financial exploitation involves taking advantage of a vulnerable individual, such as an elderly person or someone with cognitive impairments, for personal financial gain. This can include misuse of funds, manipulation, or deception.

Forgery - Forgery involves the unauthorised signing or altering of documents, signatures, or checks for fraudulent purposes, including identity fraud

Misuse of Power of Attorney - This occurs when someone with power of attorney abuses their authority to manage another person's finances by using the funds for personal benefit instead of the intended purpose.

Financial Neglect - Financial neglect occurs when a caregiver or responsible party fails to meet the financial needs of a dependent or vulnerable individual, such as neglecting to provide for basic necessities or mismanaging funds entrusted to them.

These types of financial abuse can occur independently or in combination, and they can have severe consequences for victims, including financial hardship, loss of assets, compromised financial security, and emotional distress. It's essential to recognize the signs of financial abuse and take steps to prevent and address it to protect individuals' financial well-being and security.

Recognizing the signs of financial abuse is crucial for identifying and assisting potential victims. Some tell-tale signs that someone may be experiencing financial abuse include:

- Unexplained Financial Transactions: Sudden or unexplained withdrawals, transfers, or expenditures from the victim's accounts, especially if they are large or out of character.
- Loss of Control Over Finances: The victim may exhibit a sudden loss of control over their financial affairs, such as being denied access to bank accounts, credit cards, or financial statements.
- Changes in Banking Practices: Abrupt changes in banking practices, such as frequent cash withdrawals, changes in beneficiaries, or new accounts opened without the victim's knowledge or consent.
- Significant Changes in Lifestyle: Noticeable changes in the victim's lifestyle, standard of living, or financial circumstances that cannot be explained by legitimate factors, such as job loss or medical expenses.
- Isolation or Dependency: The victim may become increasingly isolated from friends, family, or support networks, or they may exhibit signs of dependency on the perpetrator for financial assistance or decision-making.
- Signs of Coercion or Control: Evidence of coercion, manipulation, or control over the victim's financial decisions or resources by another person, such as threats, intimidation, or emotional manipulation.
- Unpaid Bills or Debt: Unpaid bills, utilities being shut off, or notices of overdue payments despite the victim having sufficient resources to cover expenses.
- Unexplained Signatures or Authorizations: Forged signatures on financial documents, changes to legal documents, or authorizations for financial transactions that the victim claims not to have made.

- Fear or Anxiety About Finances: The victim may express feelings of fear, anxiety, or confusion about their financial situation, particularly if they are unable to account for missing funds or discrepancies in their accounts.
- Reluctance to Discuss Finances: Avoidance or reluctance to discuss financial matters or seek help, even when prompted or offered assistance by trusted individuals or professionals.
- Recognizing these signs and intervening promptly can help protect potential victims of financial abuse and provide them with the support and assistance they need to regain control over their finances and well-being. It's essential to approach suspicions with sensitivity and to offer support and resources in a non-judgmental manner.

If you suspect that someone is a victim of financial abuse, there are several ways you can offer support and assistance. First and foremost, listen to the individual without judgement and let them know that you are there to help and support them. Encourage them to talk about their concerns and experiences, and reassure them that they are not alone. Offer practical assistance, such as helping them review their financial documents, budgeting, or contacting financial institutions to report suspicious activity or unauthorised transactions.

Provide information about available resources and support services, such as helplines (below), advocacy organisations, or legal aid clinics, where they can seek advice and assistance from professionals trained in dealing with financial abuse. Encourage the individual to prioritise their safety and well-being and offer to accompany them to seek help if needed. Finally, respect the individual's autonomy and decisions, and continue to offer your support and encouragement as they navigate their situation and seek assistance.

External Help:

The Financial Support Line for Victims of Domestic Abuse - 08081968845

Citizens Advice Bureau 0800 367 222 (For Scotland please call 0800 028 1456)

<u>**Honour Based Violence & Abuse**</u>

Honour-based violence and abuse (HBVA) is a deeply entrenched form of gender-based violence that persists in many cultures and societies worldwide. Rooted in patriarchal notions of family honour, HBVA encompasses a range of harmful practices perpetrated against individuals, primarily women and girls, who are perceived to have brought shame or dishonour to their family or community.

These practices may include physical violence, emotional abuse, forced marriage, female genital mutilation, and even murder, all carried out in the name of preserving family honour. Despite efforts to combat HBVA, it continues to pose a significant threat to the safety, autonomy, and dignity of individuals, often underreported and inadequately addressed within both domestic and international frameworks. Understanding the complexities of HBVA is crucial in developing effective prevention strategies, supporting survivors, and challenging the cultural norms and attitudes that perpetuate this form of violence.

Forced Marriage.

Forced marriage and arranged marriage are two distinct practices with significant differences in their nature, consent, and implications for individuals involved. An arranged marriage is a cultural or traditional practice in which families or third parties facilitate the union of two individuals, typically based on factors such as compatibility, family background, and shared values. In an arranged marriage, individuals have the autonomy to accept or decline the proposed match, and their consent is generally sought and respected throughout the process. While arranged marriages may involve familial influence or matchmaking, they prioritise the mutual agreement and agency of both parties involved, allowing them to make an informed decision about entering into the marital union.

In contrast, forced marriage involves coercion, pressure, or duress to compel one or both parties to marry against their will. In a forced marriage, individuals are denied the freedom to choose their partner or refuse the marriage, and their consent is either disregarded or obtained through threats, manipulation, or emotional blackmail. Forced marriages may occur for various reasons, including cultural expectations, familial honour, economic considerations, or perceived social obligations. Victims of forced marriage often experience severe emotional distress, loss of autonomy, and violations of their fundamental human rights.

The key distinction between arranged and forced marriage lies in the presence or absence of free and informed consent from both parties. Arranged marriages prioritise the voluntary agreement of individuals, allowing them to participate in the decision-making process and exercise their agency in choosing their life partner. In contrast, forced marriages disregard consent and autonomy, coercing individuals into marital unions against their wishes and violating their fundamental rights to self-determination and freedom of choice.

It is crucial to acknowledge that within the context of forced marriage, individuals may be coerced into unions without their consent, yet families may misrepresent such instances as arranged marriages. However, it is essential to clarify that the absence of consent fundamentally distinguishes forced marriage from its arranged counterpart. Arranged marriages, by definition, entail the mutual consent and agreement of both parties involved, underscoring the importance of autonomy in the decision-making process. Conversely, in cases of forced marriage, individuals are deprived of the freedom to choose their partner or decline the marriage, rendering any assertion of consent invalid. Therefore, it is imperative to recognize and address the coercion and violation of rights inherent in forced marriages, refraining from conflating them with the culturally accepted practice of arranged marriages.

We must, as safeguarders, recognize and support victims of forced marriage as a form of gender-based violence and human rights abuse, distinct from the cultural practice of arranged marriage. Efforts to combat forced marriage require comprehensive legal frameworks, education, advocacy, and support services to empower individuals at risk, raise awareness, and challenge the societal norms and practices that perpetuate coercion and control in intimate relationships.

Female Genital Mutilation (FGM)

Female genital mutilation (FGM), also known as female genital cutting or female circumcision, refers to the partial or total removal of the external female genitalia or other injury to the female genital organs for non-medical reasons. This harmful practice is often carried out on girls before puberty, although it can also occur in infants, adolescents, and adult women. FGM is typically performed for cultural, religious, or social reasons, and it is deeply entrenched in various communities around the world.

There are four classifications of FGM. These classifications provide a framework for understanding the varying degrees of harm inflicted upon girls and women who undergo FGM.

Type I - Clitoridectomy

Type I FGM involves the partial or total removal of the clitoris, which is a sensitive organ containing thousands of nerve endings and crucial for sexual arousal.

In some cases, only the clitoral hood (prepuce) is removed, while in more severe instances, the entire clitoris may be excised.

Type II - Excision

Type II FGM involves the partial or total removal of the clitoris and the labia minora, which are the inner folds of the vulva.

Additionally, the labia majora (outer folds) may be trimmed or repositioned, and the vaginal opening may be narrowed through stitching, leaving a small opening for urine and menstrual flow.

Type III - Infibulation

Type III FGM, also known as infibulation, is the most severe form and involves the removal of the clitoris, labia minora, and part or all of the labia majora.

Following excision, the remaining tissue is stitched together, leaving a narrowed vaginal opening that is often sealed with thorns, sutures, or other materials. This closure must be reopened for sexual intercourse and childbirth.

Type IV - Any other non-medical female genital alteration

Type IV FGM encompasses all other harmful procedures to the female genitalia for non-medical purposes, including pricking, piercing, scraping, or cauterization of the genital area. This category also includes any form of genital alteration that does not fit the criteria of the first three types but still constitutes harm to the individual.

FGM poses significant short-term and long-term health risks for girls and women who undergo the procedure.

Short-term health risks include:

Pain and Shock - Immediate pain and shock are common following the procedure, which can be severe and traumatic. In some instances this shock, combined with blood loss can result in death.

Bleeding - Excessive bleeding is a common complication during and after FGM, which can lead to hemorrhage and potentially life-threatening blood loss.

Infections - FGM increases the risk of infections, including urinary tract infections, wound infections, and tetanus, due to unsterile conditions and instruments used during the procedure.

Urinary Problems - Obstructed urinary flow and difficulty urinating may occur due to scarring or narrowing of the urinary opening, leading to urinary retention or frequent urinary tract infections.

Wound Healing Issues - Poor wound healing and delayed recovery may occur, particularly in cases of extensive tissue damage or severe forms of FGM.

Psychological Trauma - FGM can cause significant psychological trauma, including anxiety, depression, post-traumatic stress disorder (PTSD), and other mental health issues, resulting from the pain, violation, and loss of bodily autonomy experienced during the procedure.

Long-term health risks include:

Chronic Pain - Women who have undergone FGM may experience chronic pelvic pain, discomfort, or sensitivity in the genital area, affecting their overall quality of life.

Gynecological Problems - FGM increases the risk of gynecological complications, such as menstrual problems, painful menstruation (dysmenorrhea), and difficulty with sexual intercourse (dyspareunia).

Obstetric Complications - FGM is associated with adverse pregnancy and childbirth outcomes, including an increased risk of obstetric fistula, prolonged labor, postpartum hemorrhage, and perinatal deaths.

Sexual Dysfunction - FGM can lead to sexual difficulties and sexual dysfunction, including reduced sexual desire, arousal problems, and pain during intercourse (dyspareunia), affecting both physical and emotional intimacy.

Psychological Consequences - Long-term psychological consequences of FGM may include ongoing trauma, anxiety, depression, low self-esteem, and difficulties forming intimate relationships, resulting from the profound violation of bodily integrity and autonomy.

Reproductive Health Issues - FGM may lead to complications related to reproductive health, such as infertility, recurrent urinary tract infections, and long-term scarring and adhesions in the genital area.

Female genital mutilation has profound and lasting effects on the physical, emotional, and psychological well-being of affected individuals, highlighting the urgent need for comprehensive interventions to prevent FGM, provide medical and psychological support for survivors, and promote gender equality and human rights.

The practice of female genital mutilation (FGM) has been prohibited in the United Kingdom since 1985, marking a significant milestone in the country's efforts to combat this harmful practice. Subsequent legislative measures have strengthened the legal framework surrounding FGM prevention, including the enactment of specific provisions in 2015 criminalizing the act of taking a child overseas for the purpose of FGM.

The **Female Genital Mutilation Act 2003** is a landmark legislation in the United Kingdom aimed at prohibiting and preventing the practice of female genital mutilation (FGM). The act criminalizes all forms of FGM, regardless of where it is performed or the age of the victim. Key provisions of the act include:

The act makes it illegal to perform, assist, or facilitate FGM, whether in the UK or abroad. This includes taking a girl abroad for FGM (known as Extra-territorial FGM, or EFGM) as discussed above. Those found guilty of FGM-related offenses can face severe penalties, including imprisonment for up to 14 years, fines, or both. Additionally, aiding, abetting, counseling, or procuring FGM is also punishable under the law. By extending legal protections to prevent FGM from occurring abroad, the UK reaffirms its commitment to safeguarding the rights and well-being of girls and women, both domestically and internationally.

The act allows courts to issue Protection Orders to safeguard potential victims of FGM. These orders can include measures to protect individuals at risk, such as prohibiting travel or requiring surrender of passports. Healthcare professionals, teachers, and social workers have a duty to report known cases of FGM to the authorities. Failure to report FGM can result in disciplinary action or criminal charges.

When addressing the issue of Extra-Familial Female Genital Mutilation (EFGM), safeguarding professionals must maintain heightened vigilance, particularly regarding children who are being taken abroad for extended periods during the summer holidays. This vigilance is especially crucial when we hear the reasons for the trip being described as attending "a ceremony" or "becoming an adult". It is essential to exercise increased scrutiny when the destination is within or near the central belt of Africa, where the practice of FGM is prevalent. In these regions, the summer months coincide with what is commonly referred to as "cutting season," a period associated with an increased incidence of FGM rituals. Some cultural beliefs dictate that performing FGM at the outset of the school summer break allows sufficient time for the child to heal before returning to school, minimizing the likelihood of detection by teachers or safeguarding staff. Therefore, safeguarding professionals should not hesitate to employ professional curiosity when inquiring about a child's travel plans during the break, including the destination, duration, and purpose of the trip. By proactively addressing potential risks associated with EFGM, safeguarding practitioners play a crucial role in protecting children from harm and upholding their rights to physical integrity and well-being.

It is very important to recognize that victims of honour-based abuse and forced marriage encompass individuals of all genders, not solely girls or women. While the prevalent narrative often focuses on female victims, it is crucial to acknowledge that men are also susceptible to these forms of abuse and coercion. Gender-based violence, including honour-based abuse and forced marriage, can affect anyone, regardless of gender identity or expression.

Men who are victims of honour-based abuse and forced marriage may face unique challenges and barriers to seeking help and support. Societal expectations and stereotypes surrounding masculinity may contribute to underreporting and a lack of awareness about male victims' experiences. Additionally, cultural norms and beliefs may further stigmatise male victims and hinder their ability to disclose their abuse or seek assistance.

As such, it is essential to broaden our understanding of honour-based abuse and forced marriage to encompass all potential victims, regardless of gender. By raising awareness about the prevalence of abuse against men, providing gender-inclusive support services, and challenging harmful stereotypes and norms, we can create a more inclusive and supportive environment for all victims of honour-based abuse and forced marriage. This inclusive approach is essential in ensuring that all victims receive the help, support, and resources they need to escape abuse and rebuild their lives free from coercion and violence.

<u>**Modern Slavery**</u>

Modern slavery encompasses a range of exploitative practices in which individuals are subjected to various forms of coercion, control, and exploitation for the purpose of forced labour, sexual exploitation, or other forms of exploitation. It represents a grave violation of human rights and dignity, perpetuating cycles of abuse, inequality, and vulnerability. Unlike historical forms of slavery, modern slavery often operates in hidden or clandestine contexts, making it challenging to detect and address effectively.

One prevalent form of modern slavery is forced labour, where individuals are compelled to work under exploitative conditions through coercion, deception, or threat of violence. Victims of forced labour may be trapped in situations of debt bondage, where they are forced to work to repay a debt that is often inflated or impossible to repay. They may also be subjected to threats, physical violence, or psychological manipulation to ensure their compliance and prevent them from escaping.

Another form of modern slavery is human trafficking, which involves the recruitment, transportation, transfer, harbouring, or receipt of persons through force, fraud, or coercion for the purpose of exploitation. Victims of human trafficking may be trafficked for various forms of exploitation, including forced labour, sexual exploitation, forced marriage, or organ harvesting. Traffickers prey on vulnerable individuals, including migrants, refugees, and marginalised communities, exploiting their vulnerabilities for profit and personal gain.

Sexual exploitation is also a prevalent form of modern slavery, where individuals, predominantly women and children, are coerced or deceived into engaging in commercial sex acts against their will. Victims of sexual exploitation may be subjected to physical and psychological abuse, threats, and manipulation, perpetuating their exploitation and vulnerability.

In addition to these forms of exploitation, modern slavery can manifest in various other forms, including forced marriage, child labour, domestic servitude, and forced criminality. Victims of modern slavery come from diverse backgrounds and may be subjected to exploitation in various industries, including agriculture, construction, manufacturing, domestic work, hospitality, and the sex industry.#

Debt Bondage

Modern slavery encompasses a range of exploitative practices in which individuals are subjected to various forms of coercion, control, and exploitation for the purpose of forced labour, sexual exploitation, or other forms of exploitation. It represents a grave violation of human rights and dignity, perpetuating cycles of abuse, inequality, and vulnerability. Unlike historical forms of slavery, modern slavery often operates in hidden or clandestine contexts, making it challenging to detect and address effectively.

With forced labour, where individuals are compelled to work under exploitative conditions through coercion, deception, or threat of violence, victims may be trapped in situations of debt bondage, where they are forced to work to repay a debt that is often inflated or impossible to repay. They may also be subjected to threats, physical violence, or psychological manipulation to ensure their compliance and prevent them from escaping.

The National Referral Mechanism (NRM).

The National Referral Mechanism (NRM) is a framework established by the UK government to identify and support victims of modern slavery. It serves as a formal process for referring potential victims of modern slavery to the appropriate authorities for assessment and assistance. The NRM is designed to ensure that victims receive the support and protection they need to recover from their exploitation and rebuild their lives.

When a potential victim of modern slavery is identified, they can be referred to the NRM by a wide range of organisations and individuals, including police, immigration authorities, NGOs, healthcare professionals, social workers known as 'first responders;. Once a referral is made, the case is assessed by specially trained professionals within the NRM, who determine whether the individual is a victim of modern slavery based on specific criteria outlined in the **Modern Slavery Act 2015.**

If the individual is recognized as a victim of modern slavery, they are granted access to a range of support services and assistance tailored to their needs. This may include accommodation, financial support, legal advice, medical care, counselling, and assistance with immigration matters. The support provided through the NRM aims to address the immediate needs of survivors, ensure their safety and well-being, and empower them to recover from their exploitation and reintegrate into society.

In addition to providing support to individual survivors, the NRM also plays a crucial role in gathering data and intelligence on the prevalence and nature of modern slavery in the UK. This information helps inform government policies and strategies to prevent and combat modern slavery, improve victim identification and support services, and hold perpetrators accountable for their crimes.

The NRM serves as a vital tool in the UK's efforts to combat modern slavery by identifying victims, providing them with the support they need, and working towards the eradication of this heinous crime.

Learn to spot the signs

Recognizing the signs of modern slavery is crucial in identifying and helping potential victims. While the indicators may vary depending on the type of exploitation and the context, some common signs to look out for include:

Physical Signs.

- Evidence of physical abuse, such as bruises, cuts, or other injuries.
- Poor physical health, malnutrition, or signs of untreated medical conditions.
- Appearing unkempt or lacking appropriate clothing for the weather or work environment.

Behavioral Signs.

- Signs of fear, anxiety, or trauma, such as avoiding eye contact, appearing withdrawn, or displaying nervous behaviour.
- Signs of control or manipulation by another person, such as always being accompanied by someone else or appearing hesitant to speak freely.
- Signs of isolation or restricted freedom, such as being unable to leave a certain location or having limited access to communication devices.

Work and Living Conditions.

- Working excessively long hours without breaks or rest, often in unsafe or hazardous conditions.
- Living in cramped or overcrowded accommodation, sometimes with other workers or individuals under similar circumstances.
- Lack of control over personal identification documents, such as passports or identification cards, which may be held by another person.

Financial Signs.

- Being paid significantly below the minimum wage or not being paid at all for work performed.

- Having wages withheld or debts imposed, which are used to control or exploit the individual.
- Having limited or no access to personal finances or bank accounts.

Social and Emotional Signs.

- Signs of psychological manipulation or coercion, such as being threatened or intimidated by others.
- Appearing to be under the influence of drugs or alcohol, which may be used to control or exploit the individual.
- Expressing feelings of hopelessness, helplessness, or resignation about their situation.

Other Indicators.

- Unusual or suspicious behaviour by individuals in positions of power or authority, such as employers or landlords.
- Presence of multiple individuals living or working in the same location who display similar signs of exploitation or abuse.
- Unexplained changes in behaviour, appearance, or circumstances, particularly if accompanied by signs of distress or vulnerability.

Please remember that no single indicator is definitive proof of modern slavery, and many victims may not display obvious signs of exploitation. However, if you observe any of these signs or have concerns about someone's welfare, it's essential to report your suspicions to the appropriate authorities or seek advice from relevant organisations specialising in modern slavery and human trafficking.

Modern Slavery Support

The Gangmasters and Labour Abuse Authority - 0345 602 5020, option 1

Modern Slavery Helpline - 0800 0121 700

<u>**Discriminatory Abuse**</u>

Discriminatory abuse refers to any form of exploitation inflicted upon an individual based on their actual or perceived membership in a particular group or category (known as protected characteristics), such as race, ethnicity, nationality, religion, gender, sexual orientation, disability, or age. This type of abuse involves treating someone unfairly or unequally because of their personal characteristics or identity traits, often resulting in physical, emotional, psychological, or social harm.

Discriminatory abuse can manifest in various ways, including verbal abuse, insults, derogatory remarks, or hate speech directed at the victim's protected characteristic. It may also involve exclusion or segregation of the individual from social activities, services, or opportunities due to prejudice or bias. In some cases, discriminatory abuse may escalate to physical violence, harassment, or hate crimes targeting the victim based on their perceived differences.

This form of abuse not only violates the individual's fundamental human rights and dignity but also perpetuates systemic inequalities and social injustices within society. Victims of discriminatory abuse may experience profound emotional distress, trauma, and feelings of powerlessness, leading to long-term psychological and social consequences. Additionally, discriminatory abuse can create barriers to accessing essential services, support, and opportunities, exacerbating the victim's vulnerability and isolation.

Addressing discriminatory abuse requires a multifaceted approach that involves challenging discriminatory attitudes and behaviours, promoting diversity, equality, and inclusion, and enforcing laws and policies that prohibit discrimination and protect the rights of individuals from marginalised or vulnerable groups. It also involves providing support and assistance to victims of discriminatory abuse, empowering them to assert their rights, seek justice, and access resources for healing and recovery. By fostering a culture of respect, tolerance, and acceptance, we can work towards preventing and eliminating discriminatory abuse and creating a more equitable and inclusive society for all.

The presence of certain indicators may suggest the occurrence of discriminatory abuse:

- Restricting or discouraging visits or involvement of relatives or friends, thereby isolating individuals from their support networks.
- Substandard or overcrowded facilities, reflecting inadequate resources or neglectful management.
- Implementation of authoritarian management styles or inflexible regimes, fostering an environment of control and power imbalances.
- Displaying abusive or disrespectful attitudes towards service users, undermining their dignity and autonomy.

- Inappropriate use of restraints or coercive measures, violating the rights and freedoms of individuals.
- Disregarding the importance of dignity and privacy, evidenced by breaches in confidentiality or personal space.
- Failure to address or manage residents who exhibit abusive behaviour towards others, endangering the safety of fellow residents.
- Neglecting to provide sufficient nutrition, hydration, or assistance with eating, compromising individuals' health and well-being.
- Limiting choice and autonomy, thereby denying individuals the opportunity to make decisions and exercise independence.
- Misuse or mismanagement of medication, posing risks to individuals' health and safety.
- Neglecting to attend to individuals' dental, visual, or auditory needs, undermining their comfort and quality of life.
- Disregarding cultural, religious, or ethnic considerations, resulting in practices that are insensitive or inappropriate.
- Failing to respond promptly or effectively to reports or complaints of abuse, perpetuating a culture of impunity and silence.
- Interfering with individuals' personal correspondence or communication, impeding their ability to maintain connections and seek support.
- Disregarding individuals' preferences or needs in care planning and decision-making processes, demonstrating a lack of person-centred care and respect.

Safeguarding leads play a critical role in supporting survivors of discriminatory abuse by providing them with comprehensive assistance, advocacy, and access to essential services. Leads ensure that survivors receive immediate support and protection following the disclosure or identification of discriminatory abuse. They provide a safe and confidential space for survivors to share their experiences, express their concerns, and receive validation and reassurance.

Safeguarding leads conduct thorough assessments of survivors' needs and risks to develop personalised safety plans tailored to their specific circumstances. These plans may include measures to ensure the survivor's physical safety, secure alternative accommodation if necessary, and address any immediate medical or mental health needs. Leads connect survivors with a range of support services and resources, including counselling, legal assistance, medical care, housing support, and advocacy services. They liaise with relevant agencies and organisations to facilitate timely access to these services and ensure that survivors receive comprehensive care and assistance.

Safeguarding leads provide survivors with emotional support and validation, acknowledging the impact of discriminatory abuse on their well-being and self-esteem. They offer empathy, compassion, and non-judgmental listening, empowering survivors to express their feelings and concerns in a safe and supportive environment. Leads advocate on behalf of survivors to ensure that their rights are respected, their voices are heard, and their needs are addressed effectively. They empower survivors to make informed decisions about their recovery and pursue justice and accountability for the discrimination and abuse they have experienced.

Safeguarding leads maintain regular contact with survivors to monitor their progress, address any emerging needs or concerns, and provide ongoing support and assistance as needed. They ensure that survivors receive continuity of care and assistance throughout their recovery journey. Leads provide training and awareness-raising initiatives to staff, volunteers, and community members to prevent discriminatory abuse, recognize its signs, and respond effectively to disclosures or suspicions. They promote a culture of zero tolerance for discrimination and abuse within organisations and communities.

By providing survivors with comprehensive support, advocacy, and empowerment, safeguarding leads play a crucial role in helping survivors of discriminatory abuse rebuild their lives, recover from their experiences, and access the assistance and resources they need to heal and thrive.

<u>**Organisational Abuse**</u>

Organisational abuse refers to systemic mistreatment of individuals within institutional or organisational settings, such as care homes, hospitals, schools, prisons, or other facilities. Unlike individual acts of abuse perpetrated by specific individuals, organisational abuse involves failures or deficiencies within the structure, culture, policies, or practices of an institution that result in harm to those under its care or authority.

This form of abuse often occurs when there is a pervasive culture of indifference, neglect, or tolerance of abusive behaviour within an organisation, allowing harmful practices to persist unchecked. Organisational abuse may manifest in various forms, including neglect, physical abuse, emotional abuse, financial exploitation, or violations of individuals' rights and dignity.

Common indicators of organisational abuse may include:

Inadequate Staffing and Supervision - Organisations may fail to provide sufficient staffing levels or appropriate supervision, leading to lapses in oversight and accountability. This can result in neglect, safety hazards, or instances of abuse going unnoticed or unaddressed.

Poor Training and Support - Staff may lack adequate training, knowledge, or resources to effectively meet the needs of individuals under their care. This can contribute to substandard care, violations of individuals' rights, and instances of mistreatment or neglect.

Institutional Policies and Practices - Organisational policies or practices may prioritise efficiency, cost-saving, or bureaucratic procedures over the well-being and safety of individuals. This can result in harmful practices, such as overmedication, restraint, or seclusion, or the denial of basic rights and freedoms.

Culture of Silence or Fear - Organisations may foster a culture of silence, fear, or intimidation, where individuals are discouraged from speaking out about concerns or reporting instances of abuse or misconduct. This can create barriers to disclosure, perpetuate abuses, and undermine efforts to promote accountability and transparency.

Lack of Accountability and Oversight - Organisations may lack effective mechanisms for monitoring, reporting, and addressing instances of abuse or misconduct. This can result in a lack of accountability for perpetrators and failures to take appropriate action to protect individuals from harm.

PART TWO

COMPILING EFFICIENT AND EFFECTIVE SAFEGUARDING PROCESSES

<u>**Your Safeguarding Policy**</u>

Introduction

Robust safeguarding policies are vital for protecting vulnerable individuals, ensuring legal compliance, preventing abuse and harm, promoting trust and confidence, supporting staff and volunteers, and fostering accountability and transparency. By prioritising the development, implementation, and enforcement of effective safeguarding policies, organisations can create safer, more inclusive environments where the dignity, rights, and well-being of all individuals are upheld and respected.

As the designated safeguarding lead, you are likely to bear the responsibility for developing and maintaining your organisation's safeguarding policy. While this task may seem daunting, it doesn't have to be overwhelming. It's important to recognize that your safeguarding policy must be accessible and comprehensible to individuals who may not have expertise in safeguarding. Thus, simplicity is key when drawing up an effective policy.

There are several key points that must be addressed in your safeguarding policy, but they should be presented in a clear and concise manner. Begin by outlining the overarching principles and objectives of your safeguarding efforts, emphasising the organisation's commitment to protecting vulnerable individuals from abuse, neglect, and exploitation. Clearly define the roles and responsibilities of staff, volunteers, and other stakeholders in safeguarding, including reporting procedures and lines of accountability.

Ensure that your safeguarding policy covers essential topics such as risk assessment, prevention strategies, response protocols, and support services available to those affected by safeguarding concerns. Incorporate relevant legal and regulatory requirements, as well as industry standards and best practices, to ensure compliance and effectiveness. Provide practical guidance and resources to assist staff in recognizing signs of abuse, responding appropriately, and accessing support when needed.

When drafting your safeguarding policy, strive for clarity and brevity without sacrificing depth or comprehensiveness. Use plain language and avoid jargon or technical terminology that may be unfamiliar to non-experts. Consider using visual aids and examples to illustrate key concepts and enhance understanding. Solicit feedback from staff, service users, and other stakeholders to ensure that your safeguarding policy is user-friendly and meets their needs.

Remember that your safeguarding policy is a living document that requires regular review and updates to reflect changes in legislation, organisational practices, and emerging safeguarding risks. Schedule periodic reviews to assess the effectiveness of your safeguarding policy and make revisions as necessary to strengthen its impact and relevance. By prioritising simplicity, clarity, and accessibility, you can develop a safeguarding policy that effectively safeguards vulnerable individuals and promotes a culture of safety and well-being within your organisation.

It is considered best practice to review and update your safeguarding policy on an annual basis, at the very least. Additionally, any alterations should be implemented promptly following any changes in legislation or updates in industry guidance. Furthermore, it is essential to conduct a thorough review of your policy following a significant incident, as part of a comprehensive 'lessons learned' exercise. This process ensures that your safeguarding policy remains current, responsive, and aligned with evolving legal requirements and shared best industry practices.

What should your safeguarding policy contain?

Addressing this question specifically proves challenging, as what proves effective and appropriate within your organisation may not necessarily align with the functions and intricacies of another. Nevertheless, there are several fundamental components that a robust safeguarding policy should always encompass.

- **An introduction to your organisation** - Provide a basic overview of your organisation, detailing its purpose, functions, and role within its respective industry or sector. Subsequently, explain how the safeguarding policy integrates with the organisation's overarching strategy, emphasising its alignment with the organisation's mission, values, and objectives.

- **Signpost to legislation that your policy aligns with** - Provide an in-depth explanation of the legislative and official guidance sources considered during the drafting process of the document. Universal examples would include the Care Act, The Children Act, The Safeguarding Vulnerable Groups Act, and Working Together to Safeguard Children. Depending on the organisation's scope, additional legislation such as The Data Protection Act, Keeping Children Safe in Education, among others, may also be pertinent. To enhance accessibility, consider incorporating hyperlinks within the policy document directing readers to digital copies of the relevant legislation on official websites.

- **Signposting to other internal policies within your organisation that complement your safeguarding policy** - These may encompass a range of internal policies such as HR policies, grievance procedures, disciplinary protocols, and more. It's common for internal policies within organisations to overlap to some extent. As long as these policies do not contradict one another, it's beneficial to embrace the overlap and allow them to mutually reinforce and strengthen each other.

- **Legislative compliance** - Your policy should not only identify pertinent legislative documents but also reinforce your organisation's firm commitment to operating within their parameters and fulfilling associated obligations. It is essential to have a clear understanding of both the rationale and the methodology behind our actions, in addition to the specifics of what we intend to accomplish.

- **Clear definitions** - Precise definitions are crucial to crafting a policy that is easily comprehensible and devoid of ambiguity. It is imperative to establish accurate definitions for all elements impacted by the policy. This may encompass various aspects, such as legally defining an adult at risk or explaining the different forms of abuse that staff should remain vigilant against. By setting these definitions, the policy ensures consistency in interpretation and implementation, fostering greater clarity and effectiveness in safeguarding practices.

- **Set out your Objectives** - It's crucial to clearly articulate the purpose of the safeguarding policy and to underscore why safeguarding holds such paramount importance within your organisation. This means clearly defining the rationale behind safeguarding practices and emphasising its intrinsic value in protecting the well-being and dignity of vulnerable individuals. By stressing the significance of safeguarding, the policy sets a firm foundation for fostering a culture of safety, respect, and accountability within your workplace.

- **State your principals** - Integrating your company values and mission statement with the overarching ethos of safeguarding embodied in your policy is essential to establish a cohesive framework that guides organisational conduct and fosters a culture of safety and well-being. By aligning organisational values and the mission statement with the principles of safeguarding, you reinforce your commitment to upholding ethical standards and promoting the welfare of all individuals involved, including employees, customers, and service users. This alignment ensures that the organisation's core values, such as integrity, respect, and accountability, are not only reflected in its overarching mission but also permeate through all aspects of safeguarding practices. By doing so, you create a unified approach where it's values and safeguarding principles complement each other, reinforcing a culture where safeguarding is not just a policy but a deeply ingrained philosophy that guides decision-making and behaviour at every level. This integration underscores the importance of embedding safeguarding principles within the organisation's ethos, ensuring that ethical conduct and the protection of individuals' rights and dignity remain central to its mission and values.

- **Be clear on roles and responsibilities** - Within your policy document, it is imperative to clearly designate key individuals responsible for safeguarding within your organisation. This includes explicitly identifying yourself and the appointed safeguarding lead, as well as the individual tasked with overseeing safeguarding matters in your absence. Additionally, ensure that the policy provides clear guidance on who to contact in the event of your absence or unavailability. Moreover, it is essential to outline the relevant parties within your organisation who play crucial roles in safeguarding efforts. This encompasses specifying the contact details and responsibilities of the data protection officer and the health and safety manager. By providing this information, you facilitate swift and effective communication channels for addressing safeguarding concerns, data protection queries, and health and safety issues within your organisation.

- **Risk Assessment and Management** - Detail the operational procedures employed for conducting comprehensive risk assessments aimed at identifying potential risks of abuse or harm within the safeguarding context. This involves outlining the steps undertaken to assess various scenarios and environments for potential vulnerabilities and threats. By providing a detailed overview of these working processes and strategies, the safeguarding policy ensures a proactive approach to risk management and enhances the organisation's ability to protect vulnerable individuals effectively.

- **Prevention and Response Strategies** - Specify the safeguarding strategies and initiatives implemented to prevent abuse and create a culture of safeguarding within your organisation. This could include comprehensive staff training programs, targeted awareness-raising initiatives, and proactive safeguarding promotion campaigns. Detail how these strategies operate, including the content and format of training sessions, the dissemination methods for awareness-raising materials, and the channels utilised for promoting safeguarding messages. Highlight the necessity of these strategies by explaining their role in equipping staff with the knowledge, skills, and resources needed to recognize and respond to safeguarding concerns effectively. Stress their proactive nature in fostering a culture where safeguarding is prioritised, ensuring that all individuals feel empowered to report concerns and take appropriate action to safeguard vulnerable individuals. By providing a thorough explanation of these strategies and their significance, the safeguarding policy reinforces your organisation's commitment to creating a safe and supportive environment for all individuals involved.
- **Reporting Mechanisms** - It is extremely important to define and provide a comprehensive explanation of the procedures in place for responding to safeguarding concerns within your organisation. This entails clearly outlining the steps involved in reporting safeguarding concerns, including the designated reporting mechanisms and channels available to staff and stakeholders. Additionally, it is essential to make clear the support services and resources accessible to individuals affected by abuse, ensuring they have access to the necessary assistance and guidance. Furthermore, the safeguarding policy should expand upon the response procedures, detailing the roles and responsibilities of key personnel involved in handling safeguarding concerns. This includes specifying the actions to be taken upon receiving a report, the process for conducting internal investigations, and the measures for ensuring the safety and well-being of anyone affected.

- **Confidentiality** - Provide unequivocal and precise guidance on upholding confidentiality and respecting individuals' privacy rights, while simultaneously fulfilling legal obligations regarding information sharing and data protection. This entails clearly articulating the procedures and protocols for safeguarding sensitive information, ensuring that personal data is handled securely and in accordance with relevant legislation. Additionally, take the opportunity to provide clear instruction on the correct process and channels for sharing information with external agencies. This includes specifying the circumstances under which information may be shared, the authorised personnel responsible for facilitating such exchanges, the protocols for obtaining consent or ensuring legal justification for sharing sensitive data, and how the decision to share should be recorded.

- **Staff Training and Support** - Give a clear statement on your organisation's commitment to delivering thorough training and support to both staff and volunteers on safeguarding principles, procedures, and best practices. This involves providing detailed explanations of the content and structure of safeguarding training sessions, ensuring they cover essential topics such as recognizing signs of abuse, reporting procedures, and the organisational safeguarding policy itself. Furthermore, emphasis should be put on the importance of ongoing support and supervision to reinforce learning and ensure adherence to safeguarding protocols. Clearly outline which safeguarding training sessions are mandatory for staff and volunteers, specifying the frequency of refresher training sessions and the method for monitoring compliance. This includes detailing the intervals at which refresher training should be provided, as well as the mechanisms in place for tracking and recording completion of training requirements.
- External Reporting and Partnerships - Elaborate on the organisation's protocols for reporting safeguarding concerns to relevant authorities or regulatory bodies, such as Social Services or the Disclosure and Barring Service (DBS). This involves providing detailed guidance on the steps to be taken when escalating safeguarding concerns, including the designated channels for making reports and the information required for effective communication with external agencies. Additionally, emphasise the organisation's commitment to collaboration and networking with external agencies to enhance its safeguarding efforts. This entails fostering partnerships with relevant stakeholders and engaging in proactive communication and information sharing to further extend the organisation's safeguarding reach and effectiveness.

Risk Assessments

In safeguarding, as with other industries, a risk assessment is at its heart the most valuable weapon in your armoury. It serves as the cornerstone of proactive measures to identify and mitigate potential risks of harm or abuse to vulnerable individuals. By conducting comprehensive risk assessments, organisations can systematically evaluate their environments, practices, and interactions to identify areas of vulnerability and implement targeted interventions to minimise risks. This proactive approach not only enhances the safety and well-being of individuals but also demonstrates a commitment to proactive risk management and safeguarding effectiveness.

Safeguarding risk assessments are critically important for several reasons. Firstly, they enable organisations to identify and evaluate potential risks of harm or abuse to vulnerable individuals. By systematically assessing various aspects of their operations, environments, and interactions, organisations can pinpoint areas where individuals may be at risk and implement measures to mitigate these risks effectively. This proactive approach helps prevent instances of harm or abuse before they occur, safeguarding the well-being and rights of vulnerable individuals, clients and staff.

Furthermore, safeguarding risk assessments promote accountability and transparency within organisations. By documenting and reviewing potential risks and the corresponding mitigation strategies, we demonstrate our commitment as safeguarders to ensuring the safety and protection of vulnerable individuals. This not only fosters trust and confidence among stakeholders but also serves as a foundation for continuous improvement and learning within your organisation.

Failure to conduct safeguarding risk assessments can have serious consequences. Without identifying and addressing potential risks, we may leave vulnerable individuals exposed to harm or abuse. This not only compromises the well-being and safety of individuals but also exposes the organisation to legal, reputational, and financial risks. Additionally, the absence of risk assessments may indicate a lack of commitment to safeguarding principles and best practices, eroding trust and confidence among stakeholders and potentially damaging the organisation's reputation.

As the designated safeguarding lead, you bear the responsibility of overseeing the entirety of the risk assessment process, which commences with the inception and continual refinement of the risk assessment form. Designing this form requires meticulous attention to detail and a thorough understanding of the organisation's specific safeguarding needs. It necessitates a comprehensive evaluation of potential risks and vulnerabilities faced by the client base, encompassing various factors such as organisational practices, environmental considerations, and interactions with vulnerable individuals. Additionally, the form must be periodically reviewed and adapted to ensure its ongoing suitability and effectiveness in mitigating risks.

In addition to designing the risk assessment form, you must also make informed decisions regarding its storage and retention. This entails establishing protocols for securely storing the completed forms and associated documentation, taking into account data protection regulations and confidentiality requirements. Furthermore, you must determine the duration for which these records should be retained, balancing the need for historical documentation with the principles of data minimization and privacy protection.

Moreover, as the safeguarding lead, it is incumbent upon you to ensure that the workforce is adequately trained in the use of the risk assessment form and accompanying process. This involves providing comprehensive training sessions and resources to equip staff with the requisite knowledge and skills to effectively utilise the form and adhere to established safeguarding protocols. By fostering a culture of awareness and proficiency among the workforce, you maximise the organisation's ability to protect its client base and mitigate potential risks of harm or abuse.

Each organisation operates within its unique framework, characterised by specific setups, nuances, and working practices that influence the risk assessment process. While it is impractical to address every aspect comprehensively in this context, certain fundamental considerations can guide the development of effective risk assessments tailored to your organisation's distinct needs. As a guiding principle, a robust risk assessment should encompass the following key elements.

Scope and objectives - Begin by clearly defining the scope and objectives of the risk assessment. Determine the areas, activities, or processes within your organisation that need to be assessed for safeguarding risks. Clarify the specific goals you aim to achieve through the risk assessment.

Criteria and Framework - Develop a set of criteria and a framework to guide the risk assessment process. This may include identifying relevant legal requirements, organisational policies, and best practices related to safeguarding. Define the criteria for evaluating risks, such as the likelihood and severity of potential harm. This should be a separate document to your risk assessment forms itself, but should be easily accessible to all staff that will be tasked with completing the form.

Gather Information - Collect relevant information and data to inform the risk assessment. This may involve reviewing existing policies and procedures, conducting interviews with key stakeholders, and analysing incident reports or historical data related to safeguarding incidents. With this information you can not only develop a thorough form or input system, but also improve your ability to pre-empt risk.

Identify Potential Risks - Recognize and meticulously document the potential risks of harm or abuse that fall within the purview of the assessment. Delve into various facets that could exacerbate risks, including organisational protocols, environmental conditions, and interactions involving vulnerable individuals. Employ a systematic methodology, such as engaging in brainstorming sessions or conducting risk mapping exercises, to methodically pinpoint and classify potential risks. By adhering to a structured approach, you can comprehensively identify and categorise risks, thereby facilitating a more thorough assessment of safeguarding vulnerabilities within the organisation.

Assess Risks - Examine the risks that have been identified in depth, using the predetermined criteria and framework as a guide. Assess the likelihood and potential consequences of each risk by taking into account factors such as how frequently it may occur, the severity of harm it could cause, and the effectiveness of any existing control measures in place. Utilise qualitative or quantitative methodologies, such as employing risk matrices or scoring systems, to systematically prioritise the risks based on their relative significance. This meticulous evaluation process ensures that attention is directed towards addressing the most critical risks that pose the greatest threat to the safety and well-being of individuals within the organisation.

Develop Mitigation Strategies - Formulate comprehensive mitigation strategies aimed at tackling the risks that have been identified and diminishing their potential impact. Explore a spectrum of preventive measures, control mechanisms, and interventions that can be deployed to mitigate the likelihood or severity of harm arising from these risks. Prioritise these strategies based on their effectiveness in addressing the specific risks, feasibility of implementation within the organisation's context, and the resources required for execution. By prioritising and implementing these strategies, the organisation can proactively safeguard against potential harm and ensure the safety and well-being of those under its care.

Implement Control Measures - Execute the chosen mitigation strategies and control measures throughout your organisation's operations. Establish suitable safeguards, policies, and procedures to effectively address the identified risks, ensuring a robust framework for risk management. Disseminate information regarding these control measures to pertinent stakeholders, guaranteeing widespread awareness and adherence. By fostering a culture of awareness and compliance, the organisation can fortify its defences against potential risks and uphold its commitment to safeguarding the welfare of all individuals involved.

Monitor and Review - Consistently monitor and evaluate the efficacy of the enacted control measures. Conduct regular assessments to gauge the current status of identified risks, monitor fluctuations in risk levels over time, and appraise the effectiveness of mitigation endeavours. Remain vigilant in tracking any shifts in circumstances or the emergence of new risks that may impact the organisation's safeguarding efforts. Periodically update the risk assessment to incorporate fresh insights, revised information, or evolving circumstances, ensuring that the organisation remains responsive and adaptive to emerging threats and vulnerabilities. By embracing a dynamic and iterative approach to risk management, the organisation can enhance its capacity to safeguard against potential harm and promote a culture of continuous improvement in safeguarding practices.

Document and Communicate - Thoroughly document the outcomes of the risk assessment, capturing the identified risks, proposed mitigation strategies, and implemented control measures in detail. Effectively communicate these findings to pertinent stakeholders, including senior management, staff members, and external collaborators. Maintain accurate and up-to-date documentation, ensuring accessibility to facilitate transparency and accountability throughout the organisation. By meticulously documenting the risk assessment process and its results, the organisation can foster a culture of transparency, informed decision-making, and proactive risk management, thereby enhancing its capacity to safeguard against potential harm and promote the well-being of all individuals involved.

Provide Training and Support - Offer comprehensive training and ongoing support to both staff and volunteers regarding the intricacies of safeguarding risk assessment processes, procedures, and their corresponding responsibilities. It is imperative to ensure that all individuals engaged in the risk assessment comprehend their roles and possess the requisite knowledge and skills to actively contribute to safeguarding endeavours. By equipping them with the necessary expertise and resources, you empower them to effectively identify, assess, and address potential risks, thereby bolstering the organisation's overall safeguarding framework and promoting the well-being of those under its care.

Other considerations

Do not bear the misconception that the responsibility for developing your risk assessment process rests solely on your shoulders. Embrace the opportunity to collaborate with colleagues who possess firsthand experience working with your client base, encountering risks and their ramifications on a daily basis. This collective knowledge and insight represent an invaluable resource that you can tap into to enhance the effectiveness of your risk assessment efforts. By engaging in open dialogue and leveraging the expertise of your colleagues, you can gain valuable perspectives, identify potential blind spots, and strengthen the comprehensiveness of your risk assessment process.

<u>**Multi-Agency Working**</u>

In today's complex and interconnected world, safeguarding children and adults at risk requires a collaborative and coordinated approach across various agencies and sectors. Multi-agency working, often referred to as partnership working or collaborative practice, lies at the heart of effective safeguarding strategies. This chapter explores the concept of multi-agency working in safeguarding, highlighting its significance, principles, and practical applications.

Multi-agency working entails the collaboration and coordination of efforts between different organisations, professionals, and agencies involved in safeguarding vulnerable individuals. These may include social services, healthcare & mental healthcare providers, police, educational institutions, charities, and community groups, among others. The aim is to pool together expertise, resources, and knowledge to achieve common safeguarding goals and promote the well-being of those at risk. Multi-agency working is essential for several reasons. Firstly, it recognizes that safeguarding is a shared responsibility that cannot be effectively addressed by any single agency alone. By bringing together diverse perspectives and skill sets, multi-agency working enhances the capacity to identify, assess, and respond to safeguarding concerns comprehensively.

Secondly, multi-agency working facilitates early intervention and prevention efforts by fostering timely information sharing and joint decision-making. This proactive approach helps to identify risks and vulnerabilities at an early stage, preventing escalation and reducing the likelihood of harm. Moreover, multi-agency working promotes a holistic and person-centred approach to safeguarding, taking into account the unique needs, preferences, and circumstances of individuals. By collaborating across different sectors, agencies can provide more integrated and tailored support that addresses the complex interplay of factors contributing to vulnerability.

Additionally, multi-agency working enhances accountability and transparency in safeguarding practices. By working together, agencies can hold each other to account, share learning and best practices, and continuously improve the effectiveness of safeguarding interventions.

Networking

As you embark on your journey as a safeguarding lead, one of your foremost priorities is to establish connections with key professionals in your local community. A strategic approach involves identifying and reaching out to individuals who play pivotal roles in safeguarding across various sectors. Initiating contact via email serves as a proactive step in fostering collaborative relationships and promoting multi-agency working. The following stakeholders should be included in your outreach efforts:

Local Authority Children's and Adults Social Services Team - These teams are at the forefront of safeguarding efforts, responsible for assessing and responding to concerns about the welfare of vulnerable children and adults within the community.

Local Authority Designated Officer (LADO) - The LADO serves as a central point of contact for allegations against individuals who work with children. Establishing a connection with the LADO is crucial for effectively managing and responding to safeguarding concerns within your organisation.

Local Police Service Community Officer - Community officers play a vital role in safeguarding initiatives by liaising with local communities, schools, and organisations to address safety concerns and prevent crime. Building rapport with your local police service enhances collaboration and facilitates the sharing of information related to safeguarding issues.

Safeguarding Leads at Local Hospitals, Clinics, and Schools - These professionals are instrumental in safeguarding vulnerable individuals within their respective settings. Collaborating with safeguarding leads in healthcare facilities, educational institutions, and other community organisations fosters a cohesive approach to safeguarding across various settings.

While initiating contact with these professionals may present challenges and not all emails may elicit an immediate response, the importance of this exercise cannot be overstated. Taking the initiative to introduce yourself demonstrates your commitment to safeguarding and underscores the value you place on collaborative working practices. In proactively reaching out and initiating dialogue, you lay the foundation for productive partnerships and collective efforts aimed at promoting the safety and well-being of individuals within your community.

Sharing information.

Within the framework of multi-agency collaboration, the exchange of information stands as a linchpin for cohesive safeguarding efforts. It serves as a conduit through which professionals across various sectors share insights, observations, and concerns pertinent to the welfare of vulnerable individuals. This flow of information is integral to forming a holistic understanding of complex cases, identifying emerging risks, and devising tailored interventions that address the diverse needs of those under safeguarding purview.

However, the practice of information sharing in a multi agency context is not without its complexities and considerations. Professionals must navigate a delicate balance between the need to share relevant information and the duty to uphold principles of confidentiality, privacy, and data protection. Striking this balance requires a careful and informed approach that prioritises the rights and dignity of individuals while also safeguarding against potential harm. Legal and ethical frameworks play a pivotal role in guiding information sharing practices within multi agency settings. All involved professionals must adhere to statutory requirements, such as data protection laws and safeguarding legislation, which define the parameters for lawful and ethical information sharing. Compliance with these regulations is essential to safeguarding individuals' rights to privacy and ensuring that sensitive information is handled with due care and diligence.

Later in this book we will delve deeper into the intricacies of correct information sharing in multi-agency working. We will explore the principles underpinning ethical information sharing practices, examine the legal frameworks governing information sharing, and provide practical guidance on navigating the complexities of sharing information across organisational boundaries.

Formal multi-agency working.

In your capacity as a safeguarding professional, you may find yourself called upon to participate in formal safeguarding meetings and conferences, where critical measures are devised to mitigate risks and pivotal decisions are made concerning the welfare of children and adults at risk. While these gatherings may initially seem daunting, it is essential to approach them with confidence and a clear understanding of your role. Remember, everyone present shares a common goal: the safeguarding and well-being of vulnerable individuals.

Each participant in the meeting has an opportunity to contribute their perspectives and insights in a respectful and collaborative manner. The appointed chairperson oversees the proceedings to ensure that discussions remain focused and productive, and that all attendees have the opportunity to express their views without fear of confrontation. It is important to recognize that decisions are reached through consensus and joint decision-making, rather than being attributed to any single individual.

During the course of the meeting, participants may be invited to provide recommendations or assessments of risk levels, often using standardised scales or criteria. While addressing challenging or emotionally charged topics can be difficult, it is crucial to maintain professionalism and focus on the collective effort to safeguard individuals in need.

As you gain experience and familiarity with the process, you will likely find that attending these meetings becomes less intimidating over time. Familiarity with the format, procedures, and dynamics of such gatherings will increase your confidence and effectiveness as a participant. While some cases may present significant challenges, your growing expertise and understanding will enable you to navigate complex situations with greater ease and assurance. Remember, you are part of a team dedicated to safeguarding, and your contributions play a vital role in ensuring the well-being of those in your care.

Let's have a look at some of the meetings that you may be asked to attend;

Initial Child Protection Conference (ICPC)

An Initial Child Protection Conference (ICPC) is a crucial multi-agency meeting convened by the local authority's Children's Services department when there are concerns of significant harm to a child. The purpose of the ICPC is to assess the level of risk to the child and determine whether they require a Child Protection Plan to ensure their safety and well-being.

During the ICPC, professionals from various agencies, such as social workers, police officers, healthcare professionals, educators, and representatives from other relevant organisations, come together to share information, discuss the concerns, and make decisions regarding the child's welfare. The key steps involved in an ICPC typically include:

Information Sharing - Participants share their knowledge and observations regarding the child's situation, including any concerns about abuse or neglect, family dynamics, and the child's well-being.

Risk Assessment - The group conducts a comprehensive assessment of the risks and vulnerabilities facing the child, considering factors such as the severity of harm, the presence of protective factors, and the child's developmental needs.

Decision-Making - Based on the information presented and the outcome of the risk assessment, the group decides whether the child is at risk of significant harm and whether a Child Protection Plan is necessary to safeguard their welfare.

Child Protection Plan - If it is determined that the child requires protection, a Child Protection Plan is developed collaboratively with input from all relevant parties. This plan outlines specific actions and interventions to address the identified risks and ensure the child's safety and well-being.

Review Process - The ICPC also establishes a timeline for regular reviews of the Child Protection Plan to monitor progress, reassess risks, and make any necessary adjustments to the plan as circumstances change.

Throughout the ICPC process, the focus remains on the best interests of the child, with the aim of ensuring that they are protected from harm and provided with the support they need to thrive. The meeting is conducted in a structured and confidential manner, with an emphasis on collaboration, information sharing, and joint decision-making among all involved parties.

Section 47 Meeting

A Section 47 meeting is a pivotal stage in the safeguarding process, serving as a crucial juncture where professionals collaborate to delve into concerns raised regarding a child's safety and well-being. The meeting is typically convened by the local authority's Children's Services department in response to reports or suspicions of significant harm to a child. Also referred to as a Strategy Meeting or Strategy Discussion, its primary objective is to conduct a meticulous investigation into the alleged risks and determine whether statutory intervention is warranted to protect the child from harm.

Similar to an Initial Child Protection Conference (ICPC), the Section 47 meeting brings together a diverse array of professionals from pertinent agencies and disciplines. These may include social workers, law enforcement personnel, healthcare practitioners, educators, and representatives from other relevant organisations or services. Each participant contributes their insights, observations, and expertise to facilitate a comprehensive assessment of the situation at hand.

The overarching goal of the Section 47 meeting is to ascertain whether the threshold has been met to proceed with an ICPC. This involves evaluating the severity and immediacy of the risks facing the child, as well as considering the presence of protective factors within the family or environment. If the evidence suggests that the child is at significant risk of harm, the meeting may recommend initiating statutory intervention through the formulation of a Child Protection Plan.

However, if the assessment indicates that the concerns do not meet the criteria for an ICPC, the meeting may recommend alternative interventions or support mechanisms, such as early intervention services or family support programs. These preventive measures aim to address underlying issues, strengthen family dynamics, and mitigate potential risks before they escalate into more serious safeguarding concerns.

Child in Need (CIN) Meetings

Child in Need multi agency meetings, also known as Child in Need meetings, are convened to assess and address the needs of children who require additional support or services from Children's Services, but do not meet the threshold for child protection. These meetings bring together professionals from different agencies, such as social services, health, education, and housing, to collaborate on developing and implementing a plan to support the child and their family.

During CIN meetings, the focus is on identifying the specific needs of the child and family, assessing the level of risk or vulnerability, and determining the appropriate interventions and support services required to address these needs. The aim is to provide early intervention and preventative support to improve outcomes for the child and prevent further escalation of problems.Unlike a Child Protection Order, which is made when a child is at risk of significant harm and requires compulsory measures to safeguard their welfare, a Child in Need Order does not confer statutory powers of intervention or enforcement. Instead, it enables Children's Services to offer voluntary support and services to the child and their family to address their identified needs and promote their welfare.

Looked After Child (LAC) Reviews

A Looked After Child (LAC) review is a formal meeting held to review the care arrangements and progress of children who are in the care of the local authority. These reviews are a statutory requirement under the Children Act 1989 and are conducted at regular intervals to ensure that the needs and welfare of looked after children are being adequately met.

During a LAC review, various professionals and stakeholders involved in the care of the child, including social workers, foster carers, teachers, health professionals, and the child themselves if appropriate, come together to discuss and evaluate the child's care plan, placement, and overall well-being. The primary objective of the review is to assess whether the child's current care arrangements continue to meet their needs and promote their welfare.

Key aspects that may be addressed during a LAC review include:

Placement Stability - Evaluating the stability and suitability of the child's current placement, whether it be with foster carers, kinship carers, in a residential setting, or elsewhere.

Educational Progress - Assessing the child's educational attainment, attendance, and any additional support or interventions required to support their educational progress.

Health and Well-being - Reviewing the child's physical health, mental health, and emotional well-being, and identifying any specific needs or concerns that require attention.

Contact Arrangements - Considering the frequency and quality of contact between the child and their birth family or significant others, and any adjustments needed to ensure positive and meaningful relationships are maintained.

Participation and Voice: Ensuring that the child's views, wishes, and feelings are actively sought and considered in decision-making processes, and that they have opportunities to participate in the review process.

Following the LAC review, a written report summarising the discussions, decisions, and recommendations made during the meeting is produced. Depending on the outcomes of the review, adjustments may be made to the child's care plan, placement, or support services to better meet their evolving needs and promote their overall welfare. Additionally, any concerns or areas requiring further action or monitoring may be identified, and plans put in place to address them effectively.

MARAC

Multi-Agency Risk Assessment Conferences (MARACs) are structured meetings that bring together professionals from various agencies, such as police, social services, healthcare, housing, and voluntary organisations, to collectively assess and manage the risks posed by high-risk domestic abuse cases. MARACs are designed to facilitate information sharing, collaboration, and coordinated action to safeguard and support victims of domestic abuse, particularly those at the highest risk of harm.

MARACs are needed because domestic abuse cases often involve complex dynamics and multiple agencies may be involved in providing support or interventions to victims and their families. By convening all relevant professionals in one forum, MARACs ensure that comprehensive risk assessments are conducted, relevant information is shared, and appropriate strategies are developed to address the risks and needs of victims effectively. During a MARAC meeting, the following key activities typically occur.

Cases of high-risk abuse, referred to the MARAC by frontline agencies such as the police or social services, are presented to the attendees. Information about the victim's circumstances, history of abuse, risk factors, and any previous interventions or support provided is shared.The attendees collectively assess the level of risk posed to the victim and any children involved in the case. This involves considering various factors, such as the severity and frequency of the abuse, the presence of weapons or previous threats, the perpetrator's behaviour, and the victim's vulnerabilities.

Based on the risk assessment findings, safety plans are developed or reviewed to mitigate the identified risks and ensure the immediate safety of the victim and any children. This may involve coordinating emergency accommodation, implementing protective measures, such as non-molestation orders or injunctions, and providing ongoing support and advocacy services. Attendees discuss and coordinate the provision of support services and interventions to meet the victim's needs and address the underlying causes of the abuse. This may include referrals to specialist domestic abuse services, mental health support, housing assistance, legal advice, or substance misuse services.

Relevant information and intelligence about the perpetrator's behaviour, criminal history, or other risks are shared among the attendees to inform risk management strategies and enhance victim safety. MARACs monitor and review cases regularly to assess progress, evaluate the effectiveness of interventions, and ensure that ongoing risks are managed appropriately. Follow-up actions and responsibilities are assigned to relevant agencies to track and address any outstanding issues.

MARACs play a crucial role in coordinating a multi-agency response to domestic abuse, ensuring that victims receive the support and protection they need to escape abusive situations and rebuild their lives. By fostering collaboration and information sharing among professionals, MARACs help to improve outcomes for victims and reduce the risk of further harm.

MAPPA

Multi-Agency Public Protection Arrangements (MAPPA) meetings are structured meetings that bring together representatives from various agencies, including police, probation, prisons, local authorities, health services, and other relevant organisations, to manage and monitor the risks posed by certain offenders who present a high risk of harm to the public. MAPPA meetings are established to coordinate the supervision and management of these offenders in the community, with the primary aim of protecting the public and reducing the risk of reoffending. These are needed because certain offenders, such as those convicted of serious violent or sexual offences, pose significant risks to public safety upon release from custody or while serving community sentences. These individuals may have a history of serious offending, pose a high risk of harm to others, or present complex management needs that require close monitoring and supervision by multiple agencies.During a MAPPA meeting, the following key activities are likely to happen.

Cases of high-risk offenders subject to MAPPA arrangements are presented to the attendees. Information about the offender's criminal history, risk factors, current circumstances, and any previous interventions or risk management plan is shared. Attendees collectively assess the level of risk posed by the offender to the community, taking into account factors such as the nature and severity of the offences, the offender's behaviour and compliance with supervision requirements, and any relevant changes in circumstances.

Based on the risk assessment findings, attendees develop or review risk management plans to address the identified risks and protect the public. This may involve implementing specific measures to monitor and control the offender's behaviour, such as electronic monitoring, curfews, or restrictions on contact with certain individuals. Agencies collaborate to ensure that appropriate support and interventions are provided to address the underlying causes of the offender's behaviour and reduce the risk of reoffending. This may involve referrals to relevant services, such as substance misuse treatment, mental health support, or housing assistance.

Attendees will share relevant information and intelligence about the offender's behaviour, compliance with supervision requirements, and any emerging risks or concerns. This information sharing enables agencies to make informed decisions and take appropriate actions to manage the risks effectively. MAPPA meetings regularly review and monitor the progress of offenders subject to MAPPA arrangements to assess the effectiveness of risk management strategies, identify any changes in risk levels, and address any emerging issues or challenges. Follow-up actions and responsibilities are assigned to relevant agencies to ensure that risk management plans are implemented effectively.

SARs

Safeguarding Adults Reviews (SARs) are comprehensive inquiries conducted by local authorities or Safeguarding Adults Boards (SABs) following the death or serious harm of an adult at risk who was in receipt of care and support services, or where there are concerns about how agencies worked together to protect the individual from abuse or neglect. SARs are conducted to understand what happened, why it happened, and whether anything could have been done differently to prevent or mitigate the harm. SARs are needed to fulfil several important objectives.

SARs provide an opportunity for agencies and professionals involved in the care and support of adults at risk to reflect on their practice, identify any deficiencies or systemic issues, and learn lessons to improve safeguarding practices in the future. By examining the circumstances surrounding the case in detail, SARs aim to identify areas for improvement in service delivery, communication, collaboration, and risk management. SARs promote transparency and accountability by ensuring that the circumstances of serious incidents involving adults at risk are subject to independent review and scrutiny. By conducting a thorough and impartial inquiry, SARs help to hold agencies and professionals accountable for their actions and decisions, particularly if there are concerns about failures in safeguarding practices or professional conduct.

SARs contribute to the ongoing evaluation and enhancement of safeguarding systems and processes at both local and national levels. By analysing the effectiveness of safeguarding interventions and identifying areas for improvement, SARs help to strengthen the overall safeguarding framework and ensure that adults at risk receive appropriate protection and support.

During a Safeguarding Adults Review, the following key activities typically occur.

An independent panel or review team examines the circumstances surrounding the adult's death or serious harm, including their background, care and support arrangements, interactions with services, and any safeguarding concerns or interventions that were initiated. Relevant information and evidence, such as medical records, care assessments, safeguarding records, and witness statements, are gathered and reviewed to gain a comprehensive understanding of the case.

The panel or review team analyses the available evidence to identify any contributing factors, systemic issues, or areas of practice that may have impacted the outcome. This may involve considering the actions and decisions of individual professionals, the effectiveness of safeguarding processes, and the quality of inter-agency collaboration.

Based on their findings, the panel or review team develops a set of recommendations aimed at addressing any identified shortcomings or areas for improvement in safeguarding practice. These recommendations may cover a range of areas, such as training and development, policy and procedure review, inter-agency communication, and service provision.

Once the SAR is completed, the findings and recommendations are published in a report, which is shared with relevant stakeholders, including local authorities, safeguarding boards, care providers, and regulatory bodies. The report may also be made available to the public, subject to necessary confidentiality considerations.

PLO

The Public Law Outline (PLO) process is invoked by the Local Authority when there are significant concerns regarding a child's welfare. If these concerns persist without adequate resolution, the Local Authority may opt to seek intervention from the Court. The PLO process represents the final opportunity for parents to address these concerns and enhance their parenting before legal proceedings are instigated.

This procedural framework delineates the responsibilities of the Local Authority when contemplating court intervention through Care Orders or Supervision Orders. It's crucial to recognize that in cases of imminent harm or urgency, the decision to proceed directly to Court may be made by social workers. Typically spanning around three months, the PLO process may be extended if outstanding tasks necessitate completion.

During a PLO meeting, the Local Authority issues a "letter before proceedings" to parents, detailing primary concerns and the assistance rendered by Children's Services thus far. A meeting is scheduled wherein the Local Authority Solicitor, Team Manager, Social Worker, parents, and their legal representatives convene. The Team Manager elucidates the rationale behind initiating the PLO process and outlines available support from Social Care.

Social Care reviews concerns outlined in the letter to parents and provides updates on ongoing developments. Parents are afforded an opportunity to respond during the meeting. Social Care often seeks parental agreement on a document known as a 'Written Agreement,' delineating expectations and mutual commitments. Though not legally binding, breaching this agreement may prompt escalated measures from the Local Authority. Notably, Social Care is obligated to furnish parents with relevant support.

Additionally, ample time is provided during the meeting for parents to discuss the terms of any written agreement outside formal proceedings, ensuring mutual understanding and agreement before signing. Subsequent meetings are scheduled for reviewing progress and determining the necessity of continuing the Public Law Outline process.

Serious Case Reviews

Serious Case Reviews (SCRs) are initiated in response to significant safeguarding incidents or instances where there have been serious failures in safeguarding practice. These reviews are conducted to thoroughly examine the circumstances surrounding the incident, identify any systemic issues or shortcomings in safeguarding provision, and ascertain what lessons can be learned to prevent similar incidents in the future. SCRs are a critical mechanism for promoting accountability, transparency, and continuous improvement within the safeguarding system. They provide an opportunity to analyse the complexities of safeguarding cases, assess the effectiveness of interventions, and recommend measures to enhance safeguarding practice and protect vulnerable individuals from harm.

Through a detailed examination of the events leading up to the incident, as well as the responses of relevant agencies and professionals, SCRs aim to identify areas for improvement in policy, procedure, training, and inter-agency collaboration. By disseminating the findings and recommendations of SCRs to relevant stakeholders, including local authorities, safeguarding boards, and frontline practitioners, these reviews facilitate shared learning and contribute to the ongoing development of effective safeguarding systems. Ultimately, the primary goal of SCRs is to safeguard vulnerable individuals and ensure that safeguarding practices are robust, responsive, and capable of preventing future instances of harm or neglect.

Engaging with Parents and Guardians

Engaging with parents and guardians is a fundamental aspect of effective safeguarding practice. As they are in most cases the primary carers, they play a crucial role in protecting and promoting the well-being of children and in some cases adults at risk. Recognizing the importance of building trust, fostering positive relationships, and involving families in safeguarding processes, we can explore various approaches and techniques for engaging with parents and guardians in a respectful, empathetic, and culturally sensitive manner.

The role of the parent/guardian

Parents and guardians play a fundamental role in the lives of children and vulnerable individuals, both in general and within the context of safeguarding. As primary caregivers, they are responsible for nurturing, protecting, and supporting the physical, emotional, and developmental needs of their dependents. In the broader sense, parents and guardians are tasked with providing a safe and stable environment in which children can grow, learn, and thrive. This encompasses various responsibilities, including meeting basic needs such as food, shelter, and clothing, as well as fostering emotional well-being, promoting education, and instilling values and morals.

Within the realm of safeguarding, the role of parents and guardians becomes even more significant. They serve as the first line of defence in identifying and addressing potential risks or concerns that may affect the safety and welfare of their children or vulnerable family members. This involves being vigilant and proactive in recognizing signs of abuse, neglect, or exploitation, and taking appropriate action to address any safeguarding issues that may arise. Parents and guardians are also expected to collaborate with professionals and agencies involved in safeguarding, such as social workers, educators, healthcare providers, and law enforcement, to ensure that their dependents receive the necessary support and protection.

Furthermore, parents and guardians are crucial partners in safeguarding interventions and decision-making processes. They are often involved in assessments, planning meetings, and case conferences where safeguarding concerns are discussed, and decisions are made regarding the welfare and protection of their children or vulnerable family members. Their input, cooperation, and consent are essential for effective safeguarding interventions to be implemented and sustained over time. By actively participating in safeguarding processes, parents and guardians can contribute valuable insights, perspectives, and knowledge about their family dynamics, circumstances, and needs, which can inform and guide the development of tailored support plans and interventions.

In essence, the role of parents and guardians in safeguarding is multifaceted and critical to ensuring the safety, well-being, and rights of children and vulnerable individuals are upheld.

Developing a rapport with parents/guardians

Effective safeguarding practice relies on strong partnerships and open communication between professionals and parents/guardians. Building trust and rapport with parents/guardians is essential for promoting collaboration, enhancing transparency, and ensuring the well-being of vulnerable individuals. This chapter explores strategies for establishing positive relationships with parents/guardians, including the principles of active listening, empathy, and non-judgmental communication. By implementing these strategies, safeguarding professionals can foster trust, encourage cooperation, and facilitate meaningful engagement with parents/guardians in safeguarding processes.

Strategies for Building Trust and Rapport:

Active Listening - Actively listening to parents/guardians involves giving full attention to what they are saying, demonstrating empathy, and avoiding interruptions or distractions. Encourage parents/guardians to express their concerns, feelings, and perspectives openly, and validate their experiences by acknowledging their emotions and experiences.

Empathy - Show empathy towards parents/guardians by understanding and acknowledging their emotions, concerns, and challenges. Put yourself in their shoes, and strive to empathise with their experiences, struggles, and perspectives. Empathetic responses can help build rapport and strengthen the relationship between professionals and parents/guardians.

Non-Judgmental Communication - Practice non-judgmental communication by refraining from making assumptions, criticisms, or judgments about parents/guardians. Create a safe and supportive environment where parents/guardians feel comfortable expressing themselves without fear of judgement or condemnation. Focus on understanding their unique circumstances and needs, and offer support and guidance without imposing personal biases or values.

Respect and Dignity - Treat parents/guardians with respect, dignity, and sensitivity at all times. Recognize their rights as individuals and acknowledge their role as primary caregivers. Avoid patronising language or behaviour, and strive to maintain professionalism and courtesy in all interactions with parents/guardians.

Transparency - Foster transparency by providing clear and honest information about safeguarding processes, procedures, and decisions. Keep parents/guardians informed about relevant developments, updates, and outcomes, and address any questions or concerns they may have openly and transparently. Transparency builds trust and confidence in the safeguarding process and demonstrates respect for parents/guardians' rights and autonomy.

Collaboration and Partnership - Emphasise collaboration and partnership with parents/guardians as equal partners in safeguarding efforts. Involve them in decision-making processes, assessments, and planning meetings, and seek their input and involvement in developing tailored support plans and interventions. Collaborative approaches empower parents/guardians to actively participate in safeguarding processes and contribute to positive outcomes for their families.

Tips for Establishing Positive Relationships with Parents/Guardians:

- Initiate regular communication channels, such as phone calls, emails, or face-to-face meetings, to maintain ongoing contact with parents/guardians.
- Be approachable, accessible, and responsive to parents/guardians' inquiries, concerns, and requests for support.
- Demonstrate reliability and consistency in your interactions and follow-through on commitments and promises made to parents/guardians.
- Cultivate a welcoming and inclusive atmosphere where parents/guardians feel valued, respected, and accepted without judgement or discrimination.
- Seek feedback from parents/guardians about their experiences, preferences, and suggestions for improving communication and collaboration.
- Provide educational resources, guidance, and support to parents/guardians on safeguarding-related topics, such as recognizing signs of abuse, accessing support services, and promoting positive parenting practices.
- Foster a culture of trust, mutual respect, and partnership with parents/guardians by honouring their expertise, knowledge, and insights into their family dynamics and needs.

Building trust and rapport with parents/guardians is essential for effective safeguarding practice. By implementing strategies such as active listening, empathy, and non-judgmental communication, and following tips for establishing positive relationships, safeguarding professionals can strengthen partnerships, enhance transparency, and promote meaningful engagement with parents/guardians in safeguarding processes. Through collaborative efforts and mutual respect, professionals and parents/guardians can work together to ensure the safety, well-being, and rights of vulnerable individuals are upheld and protected.

Effective communication

Effective communication is paramount when discussing safeguarding concerns with parents/guardians. It requires clarity, sensitivity, and honesty to ensure that information is conveyed accurately while maintaining a supportive and respectful dialogue. This chapter provides guidance on effective communication techniques for professionals when addressing safeguarding concerns with parents/guardians. It includes strategies for fostering open and honest discussions, managing difficult conversations, and addressing resistance or defensiveness from parents/guardians.

Clarity - Use clear and concise language when discussing safeguarding concerns with parents/guardians. Avoid using jargon or technical terms that may be confusing or overwhelming. Break down complex information into understandable terms and provide examples or explanations to illustrate key points.

Sensitivity - Approach discussions with sensitivity and empathy towards the feelings and experiences of parents/guardians. Recognize the emotional impact of safeguarding concerns and acknowledge any distress or concerns expressed by parents/guardians. Be attentive to non-verbal cues, such as body language or facial expressions, and adjust your communication style accordingly.

Honesty - Maintain honesty and transparency throughout the conversation by providing accurate information and feedback. Avoid sugar coating or minimising the severity of safeguarding concerns, as this may undermine trust and credibility. Present information truthfully and openly, while emphasising your commitment to supporting the well-being of the individual or individuals involved.

Active Listening - Practice active listening by giving full attention to what parents/guardians are saying without interrupting or rushing to respond. Demonstrate empathy and understanding by validating their concerns and feelings. Paraphrase or summarise their statements to ensure mutual understanding and clarify any misunderstandings.

Respectful Language - Use respectful and non-judgmental language when discussing safeguarding concerns with parents/guardians. Avoid making assumptions or accusations that may be perceived as judgmental or confrontational. Frame discussions in a supportive and collaborative manner, focusing on solutions and constructive actions.

Empowerment - Empower parents/guardians by involving them in the decision-making process and respecting their autonomy and agency. Provide opportunities for them to voice their opinions, preferences, and concerns, and actively listen to their input. Offer information, resources, and support to help them make informed decisions about their child's well-being.

Cultural Sensitivity - Be culturally sensitive and respectful of diverse backgrounds, beliefs, and practices when communicating with parents/guardians. Recognize and accommodate cultural differences in communication styles, values, and norms, and avoid imposing your own cultural biases or assumptions.

Tips for Managing Difficult Conversations:

- Prepare in advance by gathering relevant information, clarifying objectives, and anticipating potential challenges or objections.
- Start the conversation by establishing rapport and building trust with parents/guardians through empathetic listening and respectful communication.
- Be patient and allow parents/guardians time to process information and express their thoughts and concerns.
- Use open-ended questions to encourage dialogue and exploration of different perspectives, rather than closed-ended questions that may elicit yes or no answers.
- Address resistance or defensiveness with empathy and understanding, acknowledging the validity of their feelings while gently guiding the conversation back to the main points.
- Offer reassurance and support throughout the conversation, emphasising your commitment to working collaboratively towards the best interests of the individual(s) involved.
- Summarise key points and agreements reached at the end of the conversation, and provide clear next steps or follow-up actions to maintain momentum and accountability.

Effective communication is essential for discussing safeguarding concerns with parents/guardians in a respectful, sensitive, and constructive manner. By employing techniques such as clarity, sensitivity, honesty, active listening, and cultural sensitivity, professionals can foster open and honest dialogue, build trust and rapport, and empower parents/guardians to actively participate in safeguarding processes. Additionally, by following tips for managing difficult conversations and addressing resistance or defensiveness, professionals can navigate challenging situations with professionalism, empathy, and effectiveness.

Involving parents/guardians in safeguarding

The importance of involving parents/guardians should never be underestimated the in safeguarding process. Indeed it is essential for promoting the well-being and safety of children and adults at risk. Collaborative working between professionals and parents/guardians not only enhances the effectiveness of safeguarding interventions but also ensures that the needs and preferences of families are addressed in a holistic manner. This chapter explores strategies for involving parents/guardians in safeguarding processes, discusses the benefits of collaborative working, and emphasises the importance of parental/guardian consent and cooperation in safeguarding interventions.

Strategies for Involving Parents/Guardians:

Participation in Assessments - Encourage parents/guardians to actively participate in safeguarding assessments by sharing relevant information, providing insights into the individual's strengths and needs, and expressing their concerns or preferences. Involve parents/guardians in discussions about risk factors, protective factors, and intervention strategies to ensure that their perspectives are considered in the decision-making process.

Planning Meetings - Invite parents/guardians to attend planning meetings or case conferences where safeguarding plans are developed, reviewed, or modified. Provide opportunities for parents/guardians to contribute to the development of safeguarding goals, objectives, and action plans, and collaborate with professionals to identify resources, supports, and services that meet the needs of the individual and their family.

Decision-Making Forums - Engage parents/guardians in decision-making forums where important decisions about safeguarding interventions, placements, or services are made. Foster open and transparent communication, encourage active participation, and ensure that parents/guardians have a voice in decisions that affect their family's well-being and future.

Collaborative working between professionals and parents/guardians yields numerous benefits for children and adults at risk. By involving parents/guardians in safeguarding processes, professionals can:

- Gain valuable insights into the family's dynamics, strengths, and challenges.
- Build trust and rapport with parents/guardians, leading to enhanced communication and cooperation.
- Develop holistic and individualised safeguarding plans that address the unique needs and preferences of families.
- Promote empowerment and self-efficacy among parents/guardians by involving them in decision-making and problem-solving.
- Improve outcomes for children and adults at risk by fostering a supportive and collaborative environment that prioritises their safety, well-being, and rights.

It is essential to recognize the importance of parental/guardian consent and cooperation in safeguarding interventions. Professionals should strive to obtain informed consent from parents/guardians before implementing any safeguarding measures or interventions involving their family. Respectful and collaborative communication is key to gaining parental/guardian cooperation and ensuring that safeguarding efforts are aligned with their wishes, preferences, and values. Additionally, professionals should be mindful of cultural, linguistic, and accessibility barriers that may impact parental/guardian engagement and take proactive steps to address these challenges.

Involving parents/guardians in safeguarding processes is integral to promoting the safety, well-being, and rights of children and adults at risk. By implementing strategies for collaborative working, professionals can harness the expertise, insights, and resources of parents/guardians to develop holistic and effective safeguarding plans. The benefits of collaborative working include improved outcomes for individuals and families, enhanced communication and cooperation, and empowerment of parents/guardians in safeguarding decision-making. However, it is essential to prioritise parental/guardian consent and cooperation, ensuring that safeguarding interventions are conducted with respect, sensitivity, and cultural competence.

Signposting for parents/guardians to further support

As we have established, parents/guardians play a crucial role in safeguarding the well-being of children and adults at risk. However, they may require support and access to resources to fulfil their caregiving responsibilities effectively. This chapter provides an overview of support services and resources available to parents/guardians, guidance on signposting them to appropriate support services, and emphasises the importance of offering ongoing support and reassurance throughout the safeguarding process. As a safeguarding lead you should familiarise yourself with the specific provisions available within your area.

Parenting Classes - Parenting classes offer valuable guidance, education, and skills training to parents/guardians on topics such as child development, positive discipline, communication strategies, and stress management. These classes empower parents/guardians with the knowledge and tools needed to foster healthy relationships and promote positive outcomes for their children.

Counselling Services - Counselling services provide a safe and confidential space for parents/guardians to explore their emotions, concerns, and challenges related to parenting, family dynamics, or personal issues. Professional counsellors offer support, empathy, and practical strategies to help parents/guardians navigate difficult situations, overcome obstacles, and enhance their well-being.

Advocacy Support - Advocacy support services assist parents/guardians in understanding their rights, entitlements, and options within the safeguarding system. Advocates advocate on behalf of parents/guardians, ensuring that their voices are heard, their concerns are addressed, and their rights are upheld throughout the safeguarding process.

When working with parents/guardians, it is essential to identify their support needs and provide information on relevant support services available in the community. This may include referring parents/guardians to parenting classes, counselling services, advocacy organisations, or other community-based resources. Professionals should ensure that parents/guardians have access to accurate and up-to-date information about support services, including contact details, eligibility criteria, and referral processes.

Offering ongoing support and reassurance to parents/guardians is essential for maintaining trust, engagement, and collaboration throughout the safeguarding process. Professionals should remain accessible, responsive, and empathetic to parents/guardians' needs, concerns, and questions. Regular communication, check-ins, and updates can help alleviate anxiety, clarify expectations, and reinforce the importance of working together to promote the safety and well-being of all family members.

Accessing support services and resources is vital for parents/guardians to navigate the complexities of safeguarding and fulfil their caregiving responsibilities effectively. By providing information, guidance, and signposting to appropriate support services, professionals can empower parents/guardians to access the help they need and strengthen their capacity to safeguard their families. It is crucial to offer ongoing support and reassurance to parents/guardians throughout the safeguarding process, ensuring that they feel supported, informed, and empowered to advocate for the best interests of their children and family members.

<u>**Creating a culture of safeguarding**</u>

A culture of safeguarding within an organisation is the collective mindset, attitudes, values, and behaviours that prioritise the safety, well-being, and dignity of all individuals involved. In this chapter, we will explore what constitutes a culture of safeguarding and why it is essential for ensuring the overall welfare and safety of everyone within the organisation.

A culture of safeguarding encompasses the organisational ethos that promotes an environment where safeguarding is embedded into every aspect of operations, decision-making, and interactions. It involves fostering a culture where everyone feels responsible for protecting individuals from harm, abuse, or neglect, regardless of their role or position within the organisation. This includes proactive measures to prevent harm, robust policies and procedures, effective communication channels, and a commitment to continuous improvement.

The fostering of such a culture is paramount to creating a safe, supportive, and respectful environment for all individuals within the organisation. It sends a clear message that safeguarding is a top priority and not merely a legal obligation. By embedding safeguarding principles into the organisational culture, the organisation demonstrates its commitment to upholding the rights and dignity of every individual, promoting trust and confidence among stakeholders, and safeguarding the organisation's reputation. A culture of safeguarding also serves to empower individuals to recognize and respond to safeguarding concerns promptly and effectively. It provides a framework for promoting awareness, understanding, and adherence to safeguarding policies and procedures across all levels of the organisation. Furthermore, it fosters a supportive and non-judgmental environment where individuals feel comfortable reporting concerns and seeking assistance when needed.

In addition to protecting individuals from harm, fostering a culture of safeguarding can also lead to tangible benefits for the organisation itself. By prioritising the safety and well-being of its members, the organisation can enhance employee morale, productivity, and retention. It can also mitigate the risk of reputational damage, legal liabilities, and financial losses associated with safeguarding failures.

Leadership in a culture of safeguarding

Leadership plays a pivotal role in driving and promoting a culture of safeguarding within an organisation. In this chapter, we will explore the critical role of leadership in fostering a culture of safeguarding and discuss effective strategies that leaders can employ to demonstrate their commitment to safeguarding and create an environment where safety and well-being are paramount. Leadership sets the tone for the entire organisation and shapes its values, priorities, and behaviours. By championing safeguarding initiatives and modelling appropriate conduct, leaders send a clear message that safeguarding is a top priority and non-negotiable aspect of organisational culture. Effective leadership fosters a culture where safeguarding is embedded into every aspect of operations, decision-making, and interactions.

Leaders can demonstrate their commitment to safeguarding in various ways, including:

Setting Clear Expectations - Leaders should articulate clear expectations regarding safeguarding responsibilities and behaviours, ensuring that all staff understand their roles and obligations in safeguarding individuals.

Allocating Resources - Leaders should allocate sufficient resources, including funding, staffing, and training, to support robust safeguarding practices and initiatives within the organisation.

Leading by Example - Leaders should lead by example and adhere to safeguarding policies and procedures themselves, demonstrating a commitment to upholding the organisation's values and standards.

Promoting Open Communication - Leaders should foster a culture of open communication where staff feel comfortable raising safeguarding concerns and reporting incidents without fear of reprisal or judgement.

Providing Training and Support - Leaders should prioritise safeguarding training and provide ongoing support and guidance to staff, equipping them with the knowledge and skills needed to safeguard individuals effectively.

- Regularly communicating the organisation's commitment to safeguarding through staff meetings, newsletters, and other internal communication channels.
- Conducting regular audits and reviews of safeguarding policies, procedures, and practices to identify areas for improvement and ensure compliance with legal and regulatory requirements.
- Establishing a safeguarding steering committee or working groups of key stakeholders from across the organisation to oversee safeguarding initiatives and drive continuous improvement.
- Recognizing and rewarding staff who demonstrate exemplary safeguarding practices and contribute to creating a culture of safety and well-being.

Collaborating with external partners and stakeholders, such as local authorities, regulatory bodies, and community organisations, to share best practices and enhance safeguarding outcomes at a broader level.

Effective leadership is essential for driving and promoting a culture of safeguarding within an organisation. By demonstrating commitment to safeguarding, setting clear expectations, and implementing effective strategies, leaders can create an environment where safety, well-being, and dignity are prioritised for all individuals.

Effective communication as part of a safeguarding culture

Effective communication and awareness are essential components of fostering a culture of safeguarding within an organisation. In this chapter, we will explore the critical role of communication in raising awareness about safeguarding issues, policies, and procedures. We will discuss strategies for promoting awareness among staff, volunteers, and stakeholders and explore various communication methods and platforms that can be utilised to disseminate safeguarding information effectively.

Open and transparent communication channels are vital for ensuring that all individuals within an organisation are aware of safeguarding issues and understand their role in promoting a safe environment. By promoting awareness, organisations can empower staff, volunteers, and stakeholders to recognize and respond to safeguarding concerns promptly, thereby enhancing the overall safety and well-being of individuals.

Training and Education - Offer thorough training and educational sessions covering safeguarding policies, procedures, and reporting mechanisms to all members of staff, volunteers, and stakeholders. These sessions should provide detailed information on how to recognize, respond to, and report safeguarding concerns effectively. Additionally, ensure that regular refresher training sessions are conducted to reinforce important concepts and updates, keeping all individuals informed and prepared to address safeguarding issues as they arise.

Clear Communication Channels - Implement easily accessible communication channels dedicated to addressing safeguarding concerns, which may include designated reporting hotlines, email addresses, or scheduled in-person meetings with designated safeguarding leads. These channels should be clearly communicated to all staff, volunteers, and stakeholders, ensuring that individuals feel empowered and supported to report any safeguarding issues they encounter. Additionally, provide guidance on how to use these channels effectively and assure confidentiality and anonymity for those who choose to come forward with concerns.

Staff Meetings and Workshops - Integrate discussions and workshops focused on safeguarding into routine staff meetings and training sessions to strengthen awareness and foster open dialogue surrounding safeguarding concerns. By incorporating these topics into regular gatherings, staff members can continually reinforce their understanding of safeguarding principles and practices while also providing opportunities to discuss real-world scenarios and share insights. This proactive approach not only helps to maintain a heightened level of vigilance but also promotes a culture of transparency and collaboration within the organisation.

Online Platforms - Take advantage of digital platforms including intranet portals, newsletters, and social media channels to effectively distribute safeguarding-related information and keep stakeholders informed of updates. It is imperative to prioritise accessibility and ensure that the provided information is readily available and frequently refreshed to maintain relevance. By embracing online communication channels, organisations can extend their reach and engage a broader audience, thereby reinforcing the importance of safeguarding practices and promoting ongoing awareness throughout the organisation.

Role Modeling - Set a precedent by exemplifying a steadfast dedication to safeguarding principles and cultivating an environment characterised by transparency, accountability, and openness throughout the organisation. This entails consistently modelling behaviours aligned with safeguarding values and encouraging others to adhere to these standards. By championing a culture where safeguarding is paramount, leaders instil confidence in staff and stakeholders, fostering a collective commitment to upholding the highest standards of safety and well-being for all individuals involved.

A note on delivering training and skill building

Training and capacity building are integral components of creating a safe and protective environment within any organisation. By equipping staff and volunteers with the necessary knowledge and skills, organisations can enhance their ability to identify, prevent, and respond to safeguarding concerns effectively. This chapter will explore the importance of training and capacity building in safeguarding, providing guidance on designing and implementing tailored training programs that address the unique needs of the organisation. While we will delve into safeguarding training in more detail later in this book, this chapter serves as a foundational overview of the role of training in building a culture of safety and protection.

Training plays a crucial role in ensuring that staff and volunteers are equipped with the requisite understanding and competencies to fulfil their safeguarding responsibilities. By providing comprehensive training programs, organisations can empower their workforce to recognize signs of abuse, follow established protocols and procedures, and take appropriate action to safeguard individuals under their care. Capacity building goes beyond mere training, encompassing ongoing professional development initiatives aimed at enhancing skills, fostering critical thinking, and promoting a culture of continuous learning within the workforce. Regular safeguarding training is essential for maintaining a high standard of safeguarding practice and keeping abreast of evolving risks and challenges. As safeguarding policies, legislation, and best practices evolve over time, it is imperative that staff receive regular updates and refreshers to ensure compliance and competency. By investing in ongoing training opportunities, organisations demonstrate their commitment to prioritising safeguarding and upholding the well-being of those they serve.

Designing effective safeguarding training programs requires careful consideration of the organisation's specific needs, context, and target audience. Training should be tailored to address the unique risks and vulnerabilities present within the organisation, taking into account factors such as the nature of services provided, the demographics of service users, and the organisational structure. Training content should be relevant, engaging, and accessible, incorporating a variety of instructional methods, such as presentations, case studies, role-playing exercises, and interactive discussions, to accommodate diverse learning styles and preferences.

Training and capacity building are vital components of creating a culture of safety and protection within organisations. By investing in comprehensive training programs and professional development opportunities, organisations can empower their workforce to effectively safeguard individuals from harm and ensure compliance with safeguarding policies and procedures. While this chapter provides an overview of the role of training in safeguarding, subsequent chapters will delve into specific aspects of safeguarding training in greater detail, offering practical guidance and resources for implementation.

Embedding a culture of safeguarding into policy and practice

Embedding safeguarding principles into organisational policies and practices is crucial for creating a safe and protective environment for all individuals involved with the organisation. This chapter will delve into the process of integrating safeguarding considerations into policies, procedures, and day-to-day operations. By aligning organisational practices with best practices in safeguarding, organisations can enhance their ability to prevent and respond to safeguarding concerns effectively, ultimately promoting the well-being and safety of those they serve. The integration of safeguarding principles into organisational policies and procedures is essential for ensuring consistency and coherence in safeguarding practice. Policies should clearly articulate the organisation's commitment to safeguarding, outlining the responsibilities of staff, volunteers, and stakeholders in safeguarding individuals from harm. Safeguarding considerations should be woven into various policies, including those related to recruitment and selection, code of conduct, complaints and grievances, confidentiality, risk management, and incident reporting. By embedding safeguarding principles into policies, organisations establish clear expectations and standards for safeguarding practice across all levels of the organisation.

Regular review and updating of existing policies are necessary to ensure that they remain relevant and effective in addressing emerging risks and challenges in safeguarding. Organisations should establish a systematic process for policy review, involving key stakeholders from different departments or sectors to gather feedback and insights. During the review process, policies should be assessed for alignment with current legislation, best practices, and organisational priorities. Any gaps or inconsistencies identified should be addressed through revisions or updates to ensure that policies reflect the organisation's commitment to safeguarding and promoting a culture of safety and protection. Embedding safeguarding considerations into day-to-day operations involves incorporating safeguarding principles into decision-making processes, practices, and interactions with individuals. Staff and volunteers should be trained to recognize signs of abuse, follow established protocols and procedures, and take appropriate action to safeguard individuals under their care. Regular communication, supervision, and monitoring are essential for ensuring that safeguarding practices are consistently applied and upheld across all aspects of organisational operations. By integrating safeguarding into daily routines and practices, organisations demonstrate their commitment to prioritising the safety and well-being of those they serve.

Embedding safeguarding into policies and practices is a fundamental aspect of creating a safe and protective environment within organisations. Remain mindful that by integrating safeguarding principles into policies, procedures, and day-to-day operations, organisations can establish clear expectations for safeguarding practice, enhance consistency and coherence, and promote a culture of safety and protection. Regular review and updating of policies, coupled with ongoing training and supervision, are essential for ensuring that safeguarding practices remain effective and responsive to evolving risks and challenges. Ultimately, embedding safeguarding into policies and practices demonstrates an organisation's commitment to safeguarding and upholding the rights and dignity of all individuals involved.

Monitoring and Evaluation in a Workplace Culture of Safeguarding

Monitoring and evaluation play a crucial role in ensuring the effectiveness of safeguarding initiatives within an organisation. This chapter will explore the importance of ongoing monitoring and evaluation in assessing the impact of safeguarding measures, identifying areas for improvement, and promoting continuous learning and improvement. By establishing robust monitoring and evaluation processes, organisations can enhance their capacity to create and sustain a culture of safeguarding that prioritises the well-being and safety of all individuals involved.

Monitoring and evaluation are essential components of any safeguarding program as they provide valuable insights into the effectiveness of safeguarding initiatives and practices. Through systematic monitoring and evaluation, organisations can assess the implementation of safeguarding policies and procedures, measure progress towards safeguarding goals, and identify areas of strength and weakness. By regularly reviewing and analysing safeguarding data and outcomes, organisations can make informed decisions, allocate resources effectively, and continuously improve their safeguarding practices to better protect individuals from harm.

Establishing key performance indicators (KPIs) and metrics is essential for measuring progress and assessing the impact of safeguarding initiatives. KPIs should be aligned with organisational goals and objectives related to safeguarding, such as reducing the incidence of safeguarding concerns, increasing staff awareness and knowledge of safeguarding issues, and improving response times to safeguarding incidents. Metrics should be specific, measurable, achievable, relevant, and time-bound (SMART) to ensure meaningful evaluation and comparison over time. Common KPIs and metrics related to safeguarding may include the number of safeguarding incidents reported, the timeliness of response and intervention, and the effectiveness of safeguarding training and awareness programs.

Feedback mechanisms and stakeholder engagement are integral to the continuous improvement of safeguarding practices within an organisation. By soliciting feedback from staff, volunteers, service users, and other stakeholders, organisations can gain valuable insights into their experiences with safeguarding processes and identify areas for improvement. Feedback can be collected through surveys, focus groups, suggestion boxes, or regular meetings with other safeguarding leads and representatives. Additionally, stakeholder engagement activities, such as workshops, forums, and consultation sessions, provide opportunities for collaborative problem-solving, knowledge sharing, and relationship building. By actively involving stakeholders in the monitoring and evaluation process, organisations can foster a sense of ownership, accountability, and commitment to safeguarding goals.

PART THREE

RESPONDING TO SAFEGUARDING CONCERNS

Introduction

Responding to safeguarding concerns is a critical aspect of ensuring the safety and well-being of vulnerable individuals within any organisation or community. This comprehensive guide is designed to provide safeguarding leads, professionals, and stakeholders with practical insights and strategies for effectively responding to safeguarding concerns. Whether you are a seasoned safeguarding practitioner or new to the field, this chapter will equip you with the knowledge, skills, and resources needed to navigate safeguarding challenges with confidence and competence.

Safeguarding concerns encompass a wide range of issues that may pose risks to the safety, welfare, or rights of children, adults at risk, or vulnerable individuals. These concerns can include instances of abuse, neglect, exploitation, discrimination, or other forms of harm. Recognizing and responding to safeguarding concerns requires a thorough understanding of relevant legislation, policies, and procedures, as well as effective communication and collaboration with multidisciplinary teams and stakeholders.

Timely and appropriate responses to safeguarding concerns are essential for preventing further harm, protecting individuals at risk, and promoting their well-being. Every safeguarding concern should be taken seriously and addressed promptly, with careful consideration given to the needs and circumstances of the individuals involved. Failure to respond effectively to safeguarding concerns can have serious consequences, including prolonged suffering, escalation of risks, and legal liabilities for organisations and individuals.

In responding to safeguarding concerns, several key principles should guide practice:

Safeguarding is everyone's responsibility - Responding to safeguarding concerns requires a collective effort involving all members of an organisation or community, from frontline staff to senior leaders.

Respect for dignity and rights - All responses to safeguarding concerns should be guided by principles of dignity, respect, and the promotion of individual rights.

Empowerment and participation - Individuals affected by safeguarding concerns should be empowered to participate in decision-making processes and have their voices heard.

Confidentiality and information sharing - Balancing the need for confidentiality with the duty to share information appropriately is essential for safeguarding individuals at risk.

Accountability and transparency - Clear accountability mechanisms and transparent communication processes are essential for ensuring effective safeguarding responses and learning from practice.

In the following section, we will delve into practical strategies and best practices for responding to specific types of safeguarding concerns, including abuse, neglect, exploitation, and discrimination. By applying these principles and strategies in your practice, you can contribute to creating safer, more inclusive environments where all individuals can thrive free from harm.

Principals

Responding to safeguarding concerns requires a comprehensive understanding of the principles that underpin effective practice. It is important to delve into the core principles that guide professionals in their response to safeguarding concerns, emphasising the importance of dignity, empowerment, confidentiality, accountability, and cultural competence. By adhering to these principles, safeguarding professionals can ensure that their responses are respectful, supportive, and tailored to the needs of individuals and communities.

Dignity lies at the heart of safeguarding practice, affirming the inherent worth and value of every individual. It requires treating all individuals with respect, compassion, and sensitivity, regardless of their background, circumstances, or vulnerabilities. In responding to safeguarding concerns, professionals must uphold the dignity of those affected by affirming their autonomy, privacy, and right to self-determination. This principle underscores the importance of listening to and valuing the perspectives and experiences of individuals, empowering them to participate in decisions that affect their lives.

Empowerment is essential in safeguarding practice, enabling individuals to exercise control over their lives and make informed choices about their safety and well-being. It involves promoting autonomy, agency, and self-advocacy, empowering individuals to assert their rights, voice their concerns, and access support services. Professionals must adopt a strengths-based approach, recognizing and building upon individuals' resilience, skills, and capacities. By fostering empowerment, safeguarding responses can promote independence, confidence, and self-efficacy, enabling individuals to navigate challenges and overcome adversity.

Confidentiality is a cornerstone of safeguarding practice, safeguarding individuals' privacy, and trust. It requires safeguarding professionals to handle sensitive information with discretion, ensuring that personal details are shared only on a need-to-know basis and in accordance with legal and ethical guidelines. Professionals must prioritise the privacy and confidentiality of individuals affected by safeguarding concerns, respecting their right to control the disclosure of personal information. Clear communication about confidentiality policies and procedures is essential to build trust and reassure individuals that their information will be handled confidentially and with respect.

Accountability is vital in safeguarding practice, ensuring that professionals are held responsible for their actions and decisions. It involves adherence to professional standards, codes of conduct, and legal obligations, as well as transparency and openness in decision-making processes. Professionals must be accountable to individuals affected by safeguarding concerns, providing clear explanations, feedback, and avenues for recourse. Accountability also extends to organisational systems and structures, promoting a culture of learning, improvement, and accountability across the safeguarding continuum.

Cultural competence is essential in responding to safeguarding concerns across diverse communities, acknowledging and respecting the unique cultural beliefs, values, and practices of individuals and groups. It requires safeguarding professionals to be aware of their own cultural biases and assumptions, as well as to engage in ongoing learning and reflection to enhance their cultural competence. By incorporating cultural humility, sensitivity, and responsiveness into their practice, professionals can build trust, rapport, and understanding with individuals from diverse cultural backgrounds. Cultural competence ensures that safeguarding responses are contextually appropriate, inclusive, and respectful of cultural diversity.

The principles of effective response outlined above provide a foundation for ethical, compassionate, and culturally sensitive safeguarding practice.

The Duty to Refer

In safeguarding, a duty to refer refers to the legal obligation imposed on certain professionals or agencies to report safeguarding concerns or suspicions of abuse or neglect to the appropriate authorities. This duty is typically outlined in legislation or statutory guidance and aims to ensure that individuals at risk of harm receive the necessary support and intervention.

The duty to refer is usually placed on professionals who work closely with vulnerable individuals, such as healthcare workers, social workers, teachers, and law enforcement officers. These professionals are often in a position to identify signs of abuse or neglect and are therefore required to take action to protect the individual's safety and well-being.

When professionals have reasonable grounds to believe that a child or adult is at risk of harm, they must report their concerns to the relevant safeguarding agency or authority. This may involve making a referral to children's social services, adult safeguarding teams, or the police, depending on the nature of the concern and the age of the individual involved.

Failure to comply with the duty to refer can have serious consequences, as it may result in further harm to the individual at risk and may also lead to disciplinary action against the professional or agency responsible. Therefore, it is essential for professionals to understand their legal obligations and to act promptly and appropriately when safeguarding concerns arise.

Making a referral to local authority social services.

One of the most common types of referrals that safeguarding professionals encounter involves children or adult services. While some local authorities still accept referrals via telephone, the prevailing trend is the introduction of online referral forms. These digital platforms have become the preferred method for submitting referrals, as they offer a streamlined and efficient process for collecting essential information. As such, safeguarders are often directed to complete these online forms when making referrals to children or adult services within their respective local authorities.

When there are concerns regarding a child or an adult at risk, it is vitally important that your referral meets the threshold required for acceptance and action by social services. In today's socio-political climate, local authority social services face the challenge of budget constraints and limited resources, compounded by a rapidly increasing caseload. Much akin to a job application, your referral must stand out amidst the inundation of requests for assistance. It needs to meet specific criteria, serving as a beacon of urgency and necessity.

A threshold represents a critical juncture where significant shifts occur in the circumstances or needs of a child or family. It delineates the transition points between varying levels of need and the corresponding types of services and support required. Moreover, thresholds serve as markers indicating when professionals, services, and organisations should initiate dialogue with one another and with families. This dialogue aims to comprehensively assess the situation, determine any necessary interventions, and identify potential adjustments to current approaches.

The thresholds for children's services are categorised into levels ranging from 0 to 4, each representing varying degrees of need and risk.

Level 0 - At this level, the needs and risks faced by the child are adequately addressed through universal services or by a single agency response.

Level 1 - Children classified at this level exhibit emerging issues and unmet needs that necessitate an Early Help Assessment and the possibility of a multi-agency Team Around the

Family intervention. An Early Help Plan resulting from this assessment is overseen by a trusted professional from one of the relevant agencies.

Level 2 - Children in this category have clearly identified unmet needs that require an Early Help Assessment and a subsequent multi-agency Team Around the Family response. The coordination of the resulting Early Help Plan is managed by a worker from the Early Help Service.

Level 3 (also referred to as Section 17) - Children designated at this level are considered Children in Need under Section 17 of the Children Act 1989. Their needs necessitate statutory intervention, typically involving a social worker-led Child in Need Assessment, which may culminate in the development of a Child In Need (CIN) Plan. This category encompasses children with significant and permanent disabilities.

Level 4 (also known as Section 47) - Children falling under this category are deemed to be at risk of significant harm or are currently experiencing such harm, warranting Child Protection measures under Section 47 of the Children Act 1989. This level indicates a reasonable cause to suspect that the child is suffering or is likely to suffer significant harm, triggering urgent safeguarding actions and investigations.

A good referral

To enhance the likelihood of your referral to social services being accepted, it is imperative to meet the following criteria:

For Children:

●   Provide as much relevant personal information regarding the child as possible, including their full name, address, date of birth, and details of their parents or guardians.
●   Write a comprehensive statement outlining the reasons for believing that the child has suffered or is at risk of suffering harm. This statement should include the nature and extent of the concerns.
●   Specify whether the child has any disabilities, developmental delays, or welfare needs that are likely to necessitate support services under the provisions of the Children Act 1989, with the agreement of the child's parent or guardian.
●   When concerns revolve around the possibility of Significant Harm to a child, immediate action is imperative. If there is an imminent threat to a child's safety, it is crucial to contact the police promptly by dialling 999.

For Adults:

●   Demonstrate that the adult at risk has one or more discernible care needs that require attention.
●   Show that these care needs hinder the individual from achieving two or more specified outcomes. (A list of these outcomes is provided below.)
●   Establish that the provision of assistance is necessary to prevent these care needs from adversely impacting the individual's everyday life.

Specified Outcomes

●   Managing and maintaining nutrition - The individual struggles to manage their nutrition independently, leading to risks to their health.
●   Maintaining personal hygiene - The individual faces challenges in maintaining personal hygiene, posing risks to their health or well-being.
●   Managing toilet needs - The individual experiences difficulties in managing their toilet needs independently, which may jeopardise their health or dignity.
●   Being appropriately clothed - The individual requires assistance in managing their clothing needs, affecting their health or dignity.
●   Being able to make use of the home safely: The individual encounters obstacles in utilising their home environment safely, putting them at risk of harm.

- Maintaining a habitable home environment - The individual faces difficulties in maintaining a clean and safe living environment, which may affect their health or well-being.
- Developing and maintaining family or other personal relationships: The individual struggles to develop or maintain personal relationships, leading to feelings of isolation or loneliness.
- Accessing and engaging in work, training, education, or volunteering - The individual encounters barriers in accessing opportunities for work, education, or social engagement.
- Making use of necessary facilities or services in the local community, including public transport and recreational facilities - The individual faces challenges in accessing essential community services or facilities, hindering their ability to participate in community life.
- Carrying out any caring responsibilities the individual has for a child: The individual requires support to fulfil their caring responsibilities for a child, ensuring the child's well-being and safety.
- Managing and maintaining nutrition - The individual struggles to manage their nutrition independently, leading to risks to their health.
- Engaging in recreational activities - The individual experiences difficulties in participating in recreational activities, affecting their social inclusion and well-being.

<h1 style="text-align:center"><u>Handling Disclosures</u></h1>

Handling disclosures of safeguarding concerns is a crucial aspect of the safeguarding role, requiring sensitivity, empathy, and a clear understanding of safeguarding procedures. When individuals come forward with disclosures of abuse, neglect, or other forms of harm, it is essential for safeguarders to respond promptly and effectively to ensure the safety and well-being of those involved.

As safeguarders, we must create a safe and supportive environment where individuals feel comfortable disclosing their concerns. This involves actively listening to their disclosures without judgement, providing reassurance, and offering empathy and support throughout the process. It is important to remain calm and composed, allowing the individual to express themselves freely while offering appropriate emotional support.

In addition to providing immediate support, safeguarders must also follow established safeguarding procedures for reporting and responding to disclosures. This may involve gathering relevant information, documenting the disclosure accurately, and making a referral to the appropriate authorities or support services.

Handling Disclosures from Children.

When faced with safeguarding disclosures from children reporting harm, abuse, or neglect, it is paramount to approach the situation with care and adherence to established protocols. The safety and well-being of the child are of utmost importance, necessitating a methodical and sensitive response. Below is a general guide outlining the steps to effectively handle safeguarding disclosures from children, ensuring their protection and support throughout the process.

Create a safe environment - When responding to a safeguarding disclosure from a child, creating a safe and supportive environment is crucial. Ensure that the space is safe, private, and devoid of distractions, allowing the child to feel comfortable and secure in sharing their experiences. However, it's essential to avoid conducting the conversation behind closed doors or in isolation. Instead, consider having another trusted adult present as a witness. This not only provides additional support for the child but also safeguards against any misunderstandings or misinterpretations of the conversation.

Reassurance plays a pivotal role in facilitating open communication with the child. Make it clear to them that they are in a safe place and that your primary objective is to help and support them through this process. Assure them that they are not alone and that their well-being is of paramount importance. Building trust and rapport with the child is essential for them to feel comfortable in disclosing sensitive information.

When engaging in conversation with the child, employ open-ended questions to encourage them to share their experiences freely. Avoid leading questions that may influence or bias their responses. Allow the child to express themselves in their own words, respecting their autonomy and agency in the disclosure process. By maintaining a non-directive approach, you create a supportive environment where the child feels empowered to communicate their concerns without fear of judgement or reprisal.

Listen actively - When a child comes forward with a safeguarding disclosure, active listening is paramount. Listen attentively to the child's words without interrupting or passing judgement. By providing your full attention, you convey respect for their feelings and experiences, fostering trust and openness in the conversation. Encourage the child to speak freely and express their concerns in their own words. Let them know that you are there to listen and support them, without imposing your own interpretations or assumptions.

To facilitate deeper exploration of the child's experiences, use open-ended questions that encourage them to elaborate on their thoughts and feelings. Open-ended questions invite the child to share more information and provide insights into their perspective. For example, instead of asking, "Did something happen?" you might ask, "Can you tell me more about what happened?" This approach allows the child to express themselves more fully, enabling a more comprehensive understanding of their situation. By using open-ended questions, you demonstrate a genuine interest in the child's well-being and create space for them to share their story at their own pace.

Empathic response - When a child comes forward with a safeguarding disclosure, it's essential to provide them with emotional support and reassurance. Acknowledge the courage it took for them to speak up and express their concerns. Let them know that you are there to support them through this challenging time. Reassure the child that they are in a safe environment and that their well-being is a top priority.

However, it's crucial to avoid making promises of confidentiality. Safeguarding concerns must be reported to the appropriate authorities to ensure the child's safety and well-being. Let the child know that while you are here to support them, there are certain steps that need to be taken to address their concerns effectively. Be transparent about the reporting process and assure the child that their best interests will be at the forefront of any actions taken.

Above all, assure the child that they are not to blame for what has happened. Let them know that they are not alone in dealing with the situation and that there are people who care about them and are here to help. Validate their feelings and experiences, and let them know that it's okay to feel scared, upset, or confused.

In instances where allegations of abuse or neglect arise within a home or group environment, it is incumbent upon the safeguarder to exercise professional curiosity to determine whether other children may also be affected by similar circumstances. This involves adopting a proactive approach to investigation and inquiry, seeking out additional information and clues that may indicate the presence of broader issues affecting multiple individuals.

Documenting the disclosure - Following the verbal disclosure it's crucial to document the details accurately and objectively. This includes noting down exactly what the child said, any visible injuries or signs of distress, and the date and time of the conversation. By recording this information promptly and accurately, you create a clear record of the disclosure that can be used to inform further actions and interventions.

It's essential to avoid leading questions or making assumptions about the child's experiences. Instead, allow the child to share their story in their own words and at their own pace. This ensures that the information gathered is genuine and unbiased, allowing for a more accurate assessment of the safeguarding concern.

In addition to documenting the child's words, it's also important to record any observations or behaviours that may be relevant to the safeguarding concern. This could include changes in the child's behaviour, demeanour, or appearance during the conversation. These observations can provide valuable insights into the child's well-being and help to build a more comprehensive picture of the situation. Thorough and accurate documentation is essential when handling safeguarding disclosures from children.

Follow up and referral - One crucial step in responding to safeguarding concerns is to make a referral to the local authority, as outlined in the guidance provided earlier in this chapter. This referral is an essential part of the safeguarding process, as it allows for the involvement of relevant authorities who can conduct further assessments and interventions as necessary. By following the guidance provided and making a timely and relevant referral, you can help ensure that appropriate support is provided to those in need and that safeguarding concerns are addressed effectively.

It's important to approach the referral process with care and diligence, ensuring that all relevant information is provided and that the referral is made in accordance with established protocols. This may involve gathering additional information, documenting details of the safeguarding concern, and liaising with appropriate colleagues or agencies to ensure that the referral is comprehensive and accurate.

Handling disclosures from adults at risk

Handling safeguarding disclosures from adults reporting harm, abuse, or neglect shares similarities with addressing disclosures from children, albeit with some nuanced differences. Unlike disclosures from children, adult disclosures involve complexities that require careful consideration, particularly regarding privacy and consent. The principles of safeguarding still apply, but there are additional factors to be mindful of when handling adult disclosures.

One of the key distinctions is the emphasis on respecting the autonomy and privacy of adults. While maintaining confidentiality is crucial, there are legal and ethical obligations that govern the sharing of information without consent, as outlined in the 2P principle (see section 1). This principle underscores the importance of balancing privacy rights with safeguarding responsibilities, especially when an adult's safety or well-being is at risk. Furthermore, adult disclosures may involve individuals who are more hesitant to come forward due to various reasons such as fear of retaliation, shame, or disbelief. As such, creating a safe and supportive environment becomes paramount to encourage disclosure and provide necessary assistance. It requires a delicate balance of offering support while respecting the individual's autonomy and decisions regarding the disclosure process.

In addition to privacy considerations, handling adult disclosures may also involve navigating complex emotional responses and cultural sensitivities. It requires a nuanced approach that acknowledges the individual's unique circumstances and cultural background. Empathy, active listening, and non-judgmental communication are essential skills in building trust and rapport with adults who disclose safeguarding concerns.

Ensure a Safe and Private Environment - It is crucial to create a safe and confidential space where the individual feels comfortable and secure to share their concerns. Eliminate distractions and ensure privacy to facilitate an open and honest conversation.

Respect Autonomy - Recognize and respect the individual's autonomy and right to make their own decisions. Unless there is an immediate risk to their life or safety, honour their privacy and confidentiality.

Listen Empathetically - Practice active listening by giving the individual your full attention without interrupting or passing judgement. Allow them to express themselves at their own pace, and validate their feelings and experiences.

Offer Reassurance and Support - Provide reassurance that the individual is in a safe environment and that you are there to support them. Acknowledge their bravery in coming forward and offer emotional support throughout the conversation.

Ask Open-Ended Questions - Use open-ended questions to encourage the individual to share their experiences and express their concerns freely. Avoid leading questions that may influence their responses and allow them to provide information in their own words.

Document Details - Accurately document the details of the disclosure, including what the individual said, any visible injuries or signs of abuse, and the date and time of the conversation. Maintain objectivity and record information as it is presented.

Provide Information - Inform the individual of their options and available support services, such as counselling, legal assistance, or advocacy. Empower them to make informed decisions about their next steps and provide guidance on accessing relevant resources.

Offer Ongoing Support - Offer ongoing support and follow-up to the individual throughout the safeguarding process. Keep them informed of any developments and provide assistance as needed to navigate the situation.

Respect Privacy and Dignity - Uphold the individual's privacy and dignity at all times. Refrain from disclosing sensitive information without their consent and ensure that they are treated with respect and dignity throughout the entire process.

<u>**Confidentiality and Sharing Itelligence Correctly**</u>

Confidentiality stands as a fundamental pillar within the realm of safeguarding, playing a pivotal role in safeguarding practice by protecting sensitive information while simultaneously fostering seamless communication and cooperation among professionals. Nonetheless, upholding confidentiality must be weighed against the imperative to share pertinent intelligence judiciously in order to protect individuals facing risks. In this section, we look into the bedrock principles of confidentiality, underscore the significance of correct intelligence sharing, and furnish comprehensive guidance on navigating this intricate facet of safeguarding practice. Confidentiality embodies the responsibility to guard sensitive information divulged by individuals seeking support or services, encompassing personal particulars, disclosures of abuse or harm, and other delicate data. Safeguarding professionals bear a duty to uphold confidentiality as a means to cultivate trust with individuals and honour their entitlement to privacy. This commitment serves as a cornerstone in fostering open communication and fostering an environment where individuals feel safe to disclose their concerns and seek assistance without fear of judgement or breach of trust.

The General Data Protection Regulations (GDPR) establish seven fundamental principles governing the lawful processing of personal data, emphasising the importance of upholding individuals' privacy rights. These principles provide a framework for safeguarding personal data across its entire lifecycle, from collection to destruction.

The first principle, Lawfulness, fairness, and transparency, underscores the need for processing personal data lawfully, fairly, and transparently. This involves ensuring that individuals are informed about the processing of their data, the purposes for which it is used, and their rights in relation to their data.

Purpose limitation, the second principle, emphasises the importance of processing personal data for specified, explicit, and legitimate purposes. Personal data should not be processed in a manner incompatible with these purposes, ensuring that data is not used beyond what is necessary for the intended purpose.

Data minimization, the third principle, emphasises the importance of collecting only the minimum amount of personal data necessary for the intended purpose. This principle aims to reduce the risk of privacy breaches and unauthorised access by limiting the amount of personal data processed.

Accuracy, the fourth principle, highlights the importance of ensuring the accuracy of personal data and keeping it up to date. Organisations must take reasonable steps to ensure that inaccurate or outdated data is rectified or erased promptly.

Storage limitation, the fifth principle, emphasises the need to retain personal data only for as long as necessary to fulfil the purposes for which it was collected. Organisations should establish retention periods and regularly review and delete data that is no longer needed.

Integrity and confidentiality (security), the sixth principle, underscores the importance of protecting personal data against unauthorised or unlawful processing, accidental loss, destruction, or damage. Organisations must implement appropriate technical and organisational measures to ensure the security of personal data.

Finally, Accountability, the seventh principle, requires organisations to demonstrate compliance with the GDPR and be accountable for their data processing activities. This involves maintaining records of processing activities, implementing data protection policies and measures, and conducting data protection impact assessments where necessary.

Although confidentiality serves as a cornerstone in safeguarding practice, there are instances where sharing intelligence becomes imperative to ensure the safety and well-being of individuals at risk. By sharing pertinent information with relevant agencies and professionals, safeguarding practitioners can facilitate early intervention, coordinate support services, and enable a comprehensive response to safeguarding concerns. However, it is paramount to strike a balance between safeguarding individuals and respecting their privacy rights, while also adhering to legal and ethical guidelines.

The Data Protection Act provides a framework for the responsible handling of personal data, but it is not a barrier to sharing critical information in safeguarding contexts. On the contrary, it offers guidance on how to share information lawfully and appropriately. Understanding the principles of data protection is essential for safeguarding practitioners to navigate the complexities of sharing intelligence effectively. It ensures that sensitive information is shared only when necessary and with the appropriate safeguards in place to protect individuals' privacy rights.

When determining whether to share intelligence, safeguarding practitioners must assess the level of risk and the potential impact on the individual's safety and well-being. It is essential to consider factors such as the severity of the concern, the individual's capacity to consent, and the necessity of sharing information to prevent harm or provide necessary support. By conducting a thorough risk assessment and weighing the benefits against the risks, practitioners can make informed decisions about sharing intelligence responsibly.

Furthermore, safeguarding practitioners should follow established protocols and procedures for sharing intelligence, which may include obtaining consent from the individual where possible, seeking advice from designated safeguarding leads or legal experts, and documenting the rationale for sharing information. Transparency and accountability are key principles in the sharing of intelligence, ensuring that all actions are justified, proportionate, and in the best interests of the individual's safety and well-being.

Effectively sharing intelligence in safeguarding contexts hinges upon a set of fundamental principles designed to uphold confidentiality, respect individual autonomy, and ensure the appropriate dissemination of sensitive information. These principles serve as guiding standards for safeguarding professionals to navigate the complexities of information sharing while prioritising the safety and well-being of individuals at risk.

The first principle, operating on a Need-to-Know Basis, underscores the importance of limiting the dissemination of intelligence to individuals and agencies directly involved in safeguarding or providing support services to the individual in question. By restricting access to pertinent information to only those with a legitimate need, safeguarding professionals can minimise the risk of unauthorised disclosure and maintain the integrity of sensitive data.

Informed Consent emerges as a crucial aspect of intelligence sharing, emphasising the significance of obtaining consent from the individual before divulging sensitive information to third parties. While there are exceptions where sharing may be necessary in the absence of consent, such as when there is a compelling reason to safeguard the individual or others from harm, seeking consent remains paramount to respecting individuals' privacy rights and autonomy.

Proportionality underscores the principle of sharing only the minimum amount of information necessary to achieve the safeguarding objective. This principle aims to strike a balance between safeguarding imperatives and individual privacy, ensuring that only relevant and essential information is shared while minimising the intrusion into the individual's personal affairs.

Accuracy and Reliability emphasise the importance of ensuring that any intelligence shared is based on accurate, reliable, and credible sources. Safeguarding professionals must exercise diligence in verifying the accuracy of information before sharing it, thereby mitigating the risk of disseminating misinformation or unfounded allegations that could potentially harm the individual or undermine trust in the safeguarding process.

Record Keeping serves as a foundational practice in intelligence sharing, necessitating the maintenance of clear and comprehensive records documenting the intelligence shared, the reasons for sharing, and the recipients of the information. These records not only provide a transparent account of information exchanges but also facilitate accountability and oversight in safeguarding processes.

In adhering to these principles, safeguarding professionals can navigate the complexities of intelligence sharing with diligence, integrity, and a steadfast commitment to upholding the rights and well-being of individuals at risk.

Obtaining informed consent whenever possible represents a cornerstone of ethical intelligence sharing practices, underscoring the importance of transparency and respect for individual autonomy. Whenever feasible, safeguarding professionals should seek explicit consent from the individual before disclosing sensitive information to third parties. This process involves providing a clear explanation of the purpose and potential implications of sharing the information, empowering individuals to make informed decisions about their personal data.

Prior to sharing intelligence, it is imperative to conduct a thorough assessment of the risk of harm and the necessity for intervention. This risk assessment process enables safeguarding professionals to weigh the potential benefits of sharing information against the risks posed to the individual's privacy and well-being. Consultation with colleagues or designated safeguarding leads serves as an essential safeguarding measure, providing an additional layer of scrutiny and oversight to the information-sharing process. Collaborative decision-making helps mitigate the risk of errors or oversights, ensuring that sharing is appropriate and follows established protocols. This collaborative approach fosters accountability and confidence in the safeguarding process, promoting a culture of transparency and shared responsibility.

Maintaining clear and comprehensive records of all intelligence shared is essential for accountability, transparency, and effective information management. These records should include detailed documentation of the reasons for sharing, the individuals or agencies with whom information was shared, and any relevant contextual information. Regular review and updating of information-sharing procedures are essential to ensure compliance with legal and ethical standards, as well as to adapt to evolving safeguarding requirements and best practices.

Continued support to individuals post-disclosure

Providing holistic support to individuals affected by safeguarding concerns is essential for their recovery and well-being. This approach acknowledges that safeguarding issues often have multifaceted impacts, affecting not only the individual's physical safety but also their emotional, psychological, and social well-being. By addressing these diverse needs comprehensively, safeguarding professionals can better support individuals in their journey towards healing and resilience.

Trauma-informed approaches to care and recovery are particularly crucial in safeguarding contexts, recognizing the profound impact that trauma can have on individuals' lives. These approaches prioritise empathy, validation, and empowerment, creating safe and supportive environments where individuals feel heard, understood, and respected. By acknowledging the effects of trauma and responding with sensitivity and compassion, professionals can help individuals regain a sense of control and agency in their lives.

Advocacy, counselling, and peer support services play a vital role in promoting healing and resilience among survivors of abuse or trauma. Advocates can help individuals navigate complex systems, access support services, and assert their rights, empowering them to advocate for themselves and their needs. Counselling provides a safe space for individuals to process their experiences, explore their emotions, and develop coping strategies for dealing with trauma-related symptoms. Peer support services offer the opportunity for individuals to connect with others who have had similar experiences, fostering a sense of belonging, understanding, and solidarity.

PART FOUR

TRAINING AND CONTINUOUS DEVELOPMENT

Introduction

In this section, we will explore the essential training requirements, continuing professional development opportunities, supervision and reflective practice, staying updated with changes in legislation and guidance, and personal reflection exercises tailored to safeguarding leads.

Minimum training requirements for a safeguarding lead

In the UK, the minimum training requirements to become a safeguarding lead can vary depending on the sector and organisation. However at the very least I would recommend at a minimum a Safeguarding lead should hold a level 3 qualification in child and/or adult safeguarding from a professionally recognised organisation such as the NSPCC or Educare.

Leads should undergo comprehensive safeguarding training to understand the principles, policies, and procedures related to safeguarding vulnerable individuals. This training often covers topics such as recognizing signs of abuse, responding to safeguarding concerns, and reporting procedures. Safeguarding leads should receive training specific to their sector. This may include understanding relevant legislation and guidance, as well as the duties and expectations of the safeguarding lead within their organisation.

Training on multi-agency working is important for safeguarding leads to effectively collaborate with other professionals and agencies involved in safeguarding individuals at risk. This training helps safeguarding leads understand their role within the broader safeguarding system and how to work collaboratively with partner organisations. Safeguarding leads should participate in regular refresher training to stay up-to-date with changes in legislation, best practices, and emerging safeguarding issues. Refresher training helps ensure that safeguarding leads maintain their knowledge and skills over time.

I would recommend that leads should engage in ongoing CPD activities relevant to their role and sector. This may include attending conferences, workshops, or seminars related to safeguarding, as well as pursuing additional qualifications or certifications to enhance their expertise.

Continuous Professional Development

Continuous Professional Development (CPD) is essential for safeguarding leads to stay updated on best practices, legislation, and emerging issues in safeguarding vulnerable individuals. As the landscape of safeguarding continues to evolve, safeguarding leads must actively engage in CPD activities to enhance their knowledge, skills, and competencies. This chapter explores the importance of ongoing CPD for safeguarding leads and provides guidance on accessing various CPD opportunities.

Staying abreast of developments in safeguarding is crucial for safeguarding leads to effectively fulfil their roles and responsibilities. Ongoing CPD enables safeguarding leads to remain informed about changes in legislation, policy updates, and emerging issues related to safeguarding vulnerable individuals. By participating in CPD activities, safeguarding leads can enhance their understanding of best practices, improve their ability to recognize signs of abuse or neglect, and strengthen their response to safeguarding concerns. There are numerous CPD opportunities available to safeguarding leads, ranging from workshops and seminars to conferences and online courses. Workshops and seminars provide interactive learning experiences and opportunities for safeguarding leads to engage with experts in the field. Conferences offer platforms for networking, knowledge exchange, and exposure to cutting-edge research and practices in safeguarding. Additionally, online courses provide flexibility and accessibility, allowing safeguarding leads to engage in CPD activities at their own pace and convenience.

Local authority safeguarding hubs often offer a wide array of training courses tailored to various aspects of safeguarding, available both online and through in-person sessions. To explore the available opportunities in your area, it is advisable to reach out to your local safeguarding hub directly. They can provide comprehensive information on the range of courses, workshops, and seminars offered, along with details on how to enrol or participate. In addition to local offerings, the Home Office's Virtual College website hosts a multitude of online courses related to safeguarding. These courses cover a diverse range of topics, including child protection, adult safeguarding, domestic abuse awareness, and more. Accessible from anywhere with an internet connection, online courses offer flexibility and convenience, allowing safeguarding leads to engage in learning at their own pace and on their own schedule.

By exploring the training opportunities available through both local safeguarding hubs and online platforms like Virtual College, safeguarding leads can access a wealth of resources to enhance their knowledge and skills in safeguarding. Whether through face-to-face interactions or virtual learning experiences, investing in ongoing training is essential for safeguarding leads to stay updated on best practices, legislation, and emerging issues in safeguarding vulnerable individuals. When selecting CPD opportunities, safeguarding leads should consider their professional interests, development goals, and areas for growth. It is important to choose CPD activities that align with the specific needs of the organisation and the populations served. Safeguarding leads should seek out opportunities that offer practical insights, relevant case studies, and actionable strategies for improving safeguarding practices within their respective contexts.

Supervision and Reflective Practice for Safeguarding Leads

In safeguarding roles, regular supervision and reflective practice play pivotal roles in enhancing effectiveness, ensuring accountability, and safeguarding the well-being of both professionals and the individuals they serve. This chapter explores the significance of supervision and reflective practice for safeguarding leads, offering guidance on establishing robust supervision structures and promoting reflective practices within organisations.

Supervision serves as a supportive and collaborative process wherein safeguarding leads receive guidance, feedback, and support from experienced colleagues or designated supervisors. It provides a space for safeguarding leads to discuss complex cases, seek advice on challenging situations, and reflect on their practice. Reflective practice, on the other hand, involves the systematic process of critically analysing experiences, identifying strengths and areas for improvement, and applying learning to enhance professional practice.

Regular supervision and reflective practice offer several benefits for safeguarding leads. Through supervision, safeguarding leads can gain insights, perspectives, and new strategies to address safeguarding challenges effectively. Reflective practice allows them to evaluate their approaches, learn from past experiences, and refine their practice accordingly. Supervision provides opportunities for continuous learning and professional development. It offers a platform for safeguarding leads to explore new ideas, theories, and interventions, ultimately enhancing their skills and expertise in safeguarding.

Safeguarding roles can be emotionally demanding, involving exposure to distressing situations and challenging emotions. Supervision offers a supportive space for safeguarding leads to process their feelings, alleviate stress, and prevent burnout. Regular supervision ensures that safeguarding leads adhere to professional standards, organisational policies, and legal requirements. It promotes accountability and quality assurance by monitoring practice, identifying areas for improvement, and addressing any concerns or shortcomings.

Organisations should prioritise the establishment of clear supervision structures to support safeguarding leads effectively. This may involve:

- Designating experienced professionals or designated safeguarding leads as supervisors.
- Scheduling regular supervision sessions, ensuring adequate time and resources are allocated.
- Establishing clear objectives and expectations for supervision sessions, including goals, topics for discussion, and desired outcomes.

Providing training and support to supervisors to ensure they have the necessary skills and knowledge to fulfil their role effectively.

Encouraging safeguarding leads to engage in reflective practice is essential for fostering continuous learning and improvement. Organisations can promote reflective practice by:

- Incorporating reflective activities into supervision sessions, such as case reviews, journaling, or group discussions.
- Providing resources and tools to facilitate reflection, such as reflective frameworks, self-assessment tools, or peer support networks.
- Creating a supportive culture that values learning, open dialogue, and self-awareness.
- Recognizing and celebrating instances of reflective practice and sharing success stories to inspire others.

Supervision and reflective practice are integral components of effective safeguarding practice, promoting professional development, well-being, and accountability.

Keeping abreast of legislative updates.

In safeguarding practice, staying informed about changes in legislation, policies, and guidance is paramount to ensuring compliance, promoting best practices, and safeguarding the well-being of individuals at risk. This chapter emphasises the importance of staying updated with legislative changes and provides practical strategies for safeguarding professionals to remain informed and responsive to evolving legal frameworks.

Legislation and guidance related to safeguarding are subject to regular updates and revisions to address emerging risks, enhance protections, and reflect evolving societal norms. As safeguarding professionals, it is crucial to stay informed about these changes to ensure that practice remains current, effective, and legally compliant. Failure to keep abreast of legislative updates may result in inadequate protection of individuals at risk, legal liabilities, and reputational damage to organisations.

Strategies for Staying Updated

Subscribe to Relevant Newsletters - Subscribe to newsletters from reputable organisations, government agencies, or professional bodies specialising in safeguarding. These newsletters often provide timely updates on legislative changes, policy developments, research findings, and best practice guidelines. Examples of these are the NSPCC's CASPAR mailing list for child safeguarding, and the Ann Craft Trust quarterly bulletin for adult and child safeguarding.

Join Professional Networks - Participate in professional networks, forums, or online communities focused on safeguarding. These platforms offer opportunities to exchange knowledge, share resources, and discuss emerging issues with colleagues and experts in the field. Engaging in discussions and networking activities can help safeguarding professionals stay informed about legislative updates and industry trends.

Access Online Resources - Utilise online resources such as government websites, legal databases, and professional associations' websites to access legislative texts, statutory guidance, and policy documents related to safeguarding. These resources often provide comprehensive information on legislative changes, including explanatory notes, summaries, and practical implications for practice.

Attend Training and Workshops - Participate in training sessions, workshops, or webinars focused on safeguarding legislation and compliance. These educational opportunities offer insights into legislative updates, interpretation of legal requirements, and practical strategies for implementation. Additionally, training sessions provide opportunities for interactive learning, case discussions, and networking with peers.

To effectively monitor and review changes in legislation, safeguarding professionals can adopt the following systematic approach. Assign responsibility for monitoring legislative changes to a designated individual or team within the organisation. Ensure that this responsibility is clearly defined, and sufficient time and resources are allocated for regular monitoring activities. Develop a schedule for monitoring legislative updates, taking into account the frequency of changes and the relevance to safeguarding practice. Set regular intervals for reviewing legislative texts, policy updates, and guidance documents.

Maintain comprehensive records of legislative changes, including dates of enactment, key provisions, and implications for practice. Disseminate updates to relevant stakeholders within the organisation, including safeguarding leads, frontline staff, and management teams. Evaluate the impact of legislative changes on existing policies, procedures, and safeguarding practices. Identify any gaps or areas requiring adjustments to ensure compliance with new legal requirements. Develop action plans to address any identified issues and implement necessary changes in a timely manner.

Staying updated with changes in legislation is essential for safeguarding professionals to fulfil their legal obligations, uphold best practice standards, and protect the well-being of individuals at risk

Self reflection exercises

Below are several concise yet highly beneficial exercises that a safeguarding lead can undertake as part of their self-reflection process. These exercises are designed to facilitate personal growth, enhance professional practice, and promote continual improvement in safeguarding endeavours, allowing them to reflect on their personal values and beliefs regarding safeguarding.

<u>Consider how these values influence your approach to safeguarding practice.</u>

Identify any potential conflicts between your personal values and professional responsibilities in safeguarding. Explore strategies for managing these conflicts effectively.

<u>Critical Incident Reflection:</u>

Recall a challenging safeguarding incident or situation you have encountered in your role as a safeguarding lead.

Reflect on your response to the incident, including your emotions, thoughts, and actions. Consider what went well and what could have been improved. Analyze the impact of the incident on your practice and identify any lessons learned for future situations.

Self-Assessment of Skills and Knowledge

Assess your current level of knowledge, skills, and competencies in safeguarding practice. Identify areas of strength and areas for development.

Consider how you can further enhance your skills and knowledge through training, professional development opportunities, or mentorship.

Ethical Dilemmas Reflection

Reflect on any ethical dilemmas you have encountered in your role as a safeguarding lead. Consider the competing interests, values, and principles involved.

Explore how you approached the ethical dilemma and the factors that influenced your decision-making process.

Consider alternative courses of action and reflect on the potential implications of each option.

Feedback and Self-Reflection

Seek feedback from colleagues, peers, or supervisors regarding your performance as a safeguarding lead. Consider their perspectives and insights.

Reflect on the feedback received and identify areas for improvement or areas where your strengths can be leveraged further.

Develop an action plan for addressing any identified areas for improvement and monitor your progress over time.

Cultural Competence Reflection

Reflect on your cultural competence and sensitivity in safeguarding practice. Consider how your cultural background, biases, and assumptions may influence your interactions with individuals from diverse backgrounds.

Identify strategies for enhancing your cultural competence, such as increasing your awareness of cultural differences, seeking cultural humility, and adapting your communication style to be more inclusive.

<u>Resilience and Self-Care Reflection</u>

Reflect on your levels of resilience and self-care practices in your role as a safeguarding lead. Consider the challenges and stressors you encounter and how you cope with them.

Identify any signs of burnout or compassion fatigue and explore strategies for maintaining your well-being and resilience. Consider how you can prioritise self-care activities and seek support when needed.

These personal reflection exercises are designed to promote self-awareness, self-assessment, and continuous improvement in the role of a safeguarding lead. Do not underestimate the power and value of personal reflection time. Allocate a specific timeframe within your weekly schedule to engage in these reflective exercises. While unforeseen incidents may occasionally demand immediate attention during this designated time, strive to conduct your reflection as closely as possible to the scheduled period. This consistent practice fosters regularity and ensures that reflection becomes an integral part of your routine, allowing for deeper self-awareness and professional development.

<u>**Delivering effective safeguarding training**</u>

Safeguarding training plays a critical role in equipping individuals and organisations with the knowledge, skills, and awareness necessary to protect vulnerable individuals from harm, abuse, or neglect. In today's complex and interconnected world, where safeguarding risks are ever-present, effective training is essential to ensure that individuals are equipped to recognize signs of abuse, respond appropriately to safeguarding concerns, and uphold the rights and dignity of those at risk.

The purpose of this chapter is to explore the importance of safeguarding training for both individuals and organisations involved in safeguarding practices. We will delve into the significance of continuous learning and development in safeguarding, highlighting the role of training in enhancing awareness, building capacity, and promoting a culture of vigilance and accountability. Additionally, we will discuss the relevance of this chapter to safeguarding practice, emphasising its value in guiding practitioners, educators, leaders, and other stakeholders in their efforts to create safe and supportive environments for all.

Safeguarding training is not just a legal requirement; it is a moral imperative and a fundamental aspect of responsible governance and duty of care. For individuals, such as staff, volunteers, and professionals working with vulnerable populations, safeguarding training provides essential knowledge and competencies to recognize, respond to, and report safeguarding concerns effectively. It empowers individuals to understand their roles and responsibilities in safeguarding, enabling them to contribute to the well-being and safety of those they serve.

For organisations, investing in safeguarding training demonstrates a commitment to creating safe and nurturing environments for all stakeholders, including employees, service users, clients, and members of the community. It helps organisations mitigate risks, prevent incidents of harm, and uphold legal and regulatory obligations related to safeguarding. Furthermore, by fostering a culture of safeguarding through training initiatives, organisations can strengthen trust, credibility, and reputation, thereby enhancing their overall effectiveness and impact.

In this chapter, we will delve deeper into the various aspects of safeguarding training, exploring best practices, strategies, and considerations for designing, delivering, and evaluating training programs. By understanding the importance of safeguarding training and its relevance to safeguarding practice, individuals and organisations can take proactive steps to enhance their capacity to protect and support vulnerable individuals effectively.

Understanding the background, experience, and knowledge level of training participants is paramount to the effectiveness of any safeguarding training program. Each participant brings unique perspectives, skills, and levels of familiarity with safeguarding concepts, making it essential to tailor training content and delivery methods accordingly. By acknowledging and addressing the diverse needs and preferences of participants, trainers can ensure that training sessions are engaging, relevant, and accessible to all.

Strategies for tailoring training content and delivery methods involve several key considerations. Firstly, trainers should conduct a thorough needs assessment to identify the specific learning objectives and priorities of participants. This may involve gathering information about participants' roles, responsibilities, and prior training experiences related to safeguarding. Additionally, trainers should consider the cultural, linguistic, and learning styles diversity within the group, adapting content and delivery methods to accommodate different preferences and abilities. One important aspect of tailoring training to diverse audiences is the recognition of potential sensitivities and triggers associated with safeguarding topics. Some participants may have personal experiences or strong emotional reactions to certain themes, such as abuse or trauma. In such cases, trainers should provide advance warning when sensitive topics are to be discussed and offer participants the option to step out or seek additional support if needed. Creating a safe and supportive environment where participants feel respected and understood is essential to promoting open dialogue and effective learning.

Ultimately, by taking into account the background, experience, and knowledge level of training participants, trainers can ensure that safeguarding training programs are relevant, engaging, and impactful. By tailoring content and delivery methods to suit the diverse needs of participants, trainers can maximise the effectiveness of training sessions and empower individuals to contribute effectively to safeguarding efforts within their organisations and communities.

Set clear learning objectives

Setting clear and measurable learning objectives is essential for delivering effective safeguarding training. In this chapter, we will explore the significance of establishing clear learning objectives and provide guidance on identifying specific knowledge and skills that participants should acquire by the end of the training session. Clear learning objectives serve as the foundation for effective training programs. They provide participants with a roadmap for what they can expect to learn and achieve during the training session. By clearly articulating the desired outcomes, trainers can help participants stay focused, motivated, and engaged throughout the training process. Additionally, clear learning objectives enable trainers to assess participant progress and tailor the training content and delivery methods as needed to ensure that learning goals are met.

When setting learning objectives for safeguarding training, it is important to identify specific knowledge and skills that participants should acquire. This may include understanding the signs and indicators of abuse, knowing how to respond to safeguarding concerns, and implementing safeguarding policies and procedures effectively. By breaking down the overarching goal of safeguarding training into specific learning objectives, trainers can ensure that participants develop the necessary competencies to safeguard individuals at risk effectively.

When setting learning objectives for safeguarding training, consider the following guidance:

Be Specific and Measurable - Learning objectives should be clear, specific, and measurable. Clearly define what participants should know or be able to do by the end of the training session, and use measurable criteria to assess their achievement of these objectives.

Align with Training Goals - Ensure that learning objectives align with the overall goals and purpose of the safeguarding provision within your organisation . Consider the needs and priorities of participants and the organisation when setting objectives.

Prioritise Key Areas - Identify the most critical knowledge and skills that participants need to acquire to effectively safeguard individuals at risk. Prioritise these key areas when setting learning objectives to ensure that training remains focused and relevant.

Consider Audience Needs - Tailor learning objectives to suit the background, experience, and knowledge level of participants. Consider the diverse learning styles, preferences, and abilities within the audience when setting objectives.

Review and Revise - Regularly review and revise learning objectives to ensure that they remain relevant and aligned with changing organisational needs and emerging safeguarding issues. Solicit feedback from participants to identify areas for improvement and refinement.

Setting clear learning objectives is essential for delivering effective safeguarding training. By clearly defining what participants should know or be able to do by the end of the training session, trainers can ensure that learning goals are met and that participants acquire the knowledge and skills needed to safeguard individuals at risk effectively.

Selecting appropriate training methods

Selecting the appropriate training methods is crucial for delivering effective safeguarding training. In this chapter, we will provide an overview of various training methods and techniques suitable for delivering safeguarding training. We will explore the pros and cons of each method to help trainers make informed decisions when designing and delivering training sessions.

Presentations:

Pros - Presentations are a common and straightforward method for delivering information to a large group of participants. They allow trainers to cover a wide range of topics efficiently.

Cons - Presentations can be passive and may lead to disengagement among participants. They may also lack interactivity, making it challenging for participants to apply the information to real-life scenarios.

Case Studies:

Pros - Case studies provide participants with real-life scenarios that allow them to apply theoretical knowledge to practical situations. They encourage critical thinking and problem-solving skills.

Cons - Developing relevant and realistic case studies can be time-consuming. Additionally, some participants may struggle to relate to the scenarios presented, affecting their engagement. To assist with this I have included some real life case studies in the next section.

Role-Plays:

Pros - Role-plays allow participants to practise applying safeguarding principles in simulated scenarios. They provide opportunities for active learning, skill development, and peer feedback.

Cons - Some participants may feel uncomfortable or self-conscious participating in role-plays. Trainers must create a supportive environment to encourage participation and ensure that role-plays are conducted respectfully.

Interactive Discussions:

Pros - Interactive discussions promote active engagement and encourage participants to share their perspectives, experiences, and insights. They foster collaboration, peer learning, and the exchange of ideas.

Cons - Facilitating interactive discussions requires skilled moderation to ensure that all participants have the opportunity to contribute and that discussions remain focused and productive.

When selecting training methods for safeguarding, consider the following factors:

Audience Preferences - Take into account the preferences, learning styles, and needs of participants when choosing training methods.

Training Objectives - Align training methods with the desired learning outcomes and objectives of the training session.

Time and Resources - Consider the time, resources, and logistics available for delivering training, including the size of the group, venue, and available technology.

Diversity and Inclusivity - Choose methods that accommodate the diverse backgrounds, experiences, and abilities of participants and promote inclusivity.

Selecting appropriate training methods is essential for delivering effective safeguarding training. By understanding the pros and cons of various methods, trainers can choose the most suitable approaches to engage participants, promote active learning, and achieve the desired training outcomes.

Using the right training materials

Effective training materials play a crucial role in engaging participants and enhancing their understanding of safeguarding concepts. In this chapter, we will explore strategies for creating informative and engaging training materials, including PowerPoint presentations, handouts, and multimedia resources. By incorporating real-life examples, scenarios, and visuals, trainers can effectively communicate key concepts and promote active learning among participants.

PowerPoint presentations are commonly used in training sessions to deliver information in a visually appealing format. To create engaging PowerPoint presentations for safeguarding training Use clear and concise slides with bullet points or short sentences to convey key information. Incorporate visuals such as images, graphs, and diagrams to illustrate concepts and make the presentation visually appealing. Limit the amount of text on each slide to avoid overwhelming participants and maintain their attention. Include interactive elements such as quizzes, polls, or discussion questions to encourage active participation.

Handouts are valuable resources that participants can refer to during and after the training session. When creating handouts for safeguarding training. Organise information in a logical and easy-to-follow format, using headings, bullet points, and numbered lists. Include real-life examples, case studies, or scenarios to reinforce key concepts and illustrate their practical application. Provide space for participants to take notes and jot down their thoughts or questions. Ensure that handouts are visually appealing, with clear fonts, ample white space, and relevant graphics or images.

Multimedia resources such as videos, audio clips, or interactive simulations can enhance participant engagement and comprehension. When incorporating multimedia resources into safeguarding training Choose high-quality and relevant multimedia content that aligns with the training objectives and reinforces key messages. Integrate multimedia resources strategically throughout the training session to break up the presentation and maintain participants' interest.

Provide opportunities for participants to discuss or reflect on the multimedia content, encouraging active engagement and critical thinking. Ensure that multimedia resources are accessible to all participants, including those with visual or hearing impairments, by providing captions, transcripts, or alternative formats as needed.

Ensuring Accessibility and Inclusivity in Safeguarding Training

Ensuring accessibility and inclusivity is paramount for delivering effective safeguarding training that meets the needs of all participants. In this chapter, we will explore the importance of considering accessibility and inclusivity principles when planning and delivering safeguarding training. By providing materials in alternative formats and accommodating diverse learning styles and needs, trainers can create an inclusive learning environment where all participants can fully engage and benefit from the training.

Providing Materials in Alternative Formats - Ensure that training materials, including presentations, handouts, and resources, are available in alternative formats to accommodate participants with diverse needs.

Offer materials in accessible formats such as large print, Braille, audio recordings, or electronic text to ensure that all participants can access the information effectively.

Provide options for participants to request materials in their preferred format before the training session to ensure that their needs are met.

Accommodating Diverse Learning Styles - Recognize that participants may have diverse learning styles and preferences, including visual, auditory, kinesthetic, or tactile learning. Incorporate a variety of teaching methods and techniques, such as visual aids, group discussions, hands-on activities, and role-playing exercises, to accommodate different learning styles. Allow participants to choose activities or exercises that align with their learning preferences and encourage active participation in a way that feels comfortable and engaging for them.

Creating a Welcoming and Inclusive Environment - Foster a welcoming and inclusive environment where all participants feel respected, valued, and supported.

Encourage open communication and active participation, and create opportunities for participants to share their perspectives, experiences, and concerns. Address any discriminatory behaviour or language promptly and ensure that all interactions are respectful and inclusive.

Seeking and making the best use of training evaluation.

Effective evaluation is the cornerstone for assessing the impact and success of safeguarding training initiatives. In this chapter, we will explore various methods for evaluating the effectiveness of safeguarding training programs. By using pre- and post-training assessments, participant feedback surveys, and observation of skill demonstrations, trainers can gather valuable insights into the training's strengths and areas for improvement. Additionally, we will discuss the importance of using evaluation findings to inform future training improvements and adjustments, ultimately enhancing the quality and impact of safeguarding education.

Pre- and Post-Training Assessments - Conducting pre- and post-training assessments allows trainers to measure participants' knowledge, skills, and attitudes before and after completing the training. Pre-training assessments provide baseline data to identify participants' existing knowledge gaps and areas for improvement. Post-training assessments measure the effectiveness of the training in addressing learning objectives and enhancing participants' understanding and competencies in safeguarding practices.

Participant Feedback Surveys - Administering participant feedback surveys gathers insights from participants about their training experience, including the content, delivery methods, and overall satisfaction. Feedback surveys should include both quantitative rating scales and open-ended questions to capture participants' opinions, suggestions, and areas of concern. Analysing feedback survey data allows trainers to identify strengths and weaknesses in the training program and make targeted improvements based on participants' feedback.

Observation of Skill Demonstrations - Observing participants' skill demonstrations during training sessions provides valuable information about their ability to apply safeguarding concepts and techniques in practice.

Trainers can use structured observation checklists to assess participants' performance and identify areas for skill development or refinement. Feedback and coaching provided during skill demonstrations help reinforce learning and support participants' professional growth and development.

Identifying Strengths and Areas for Improvement - Analysing evaluation data allows trainers to identify training strengths and areas for improvement based on participants' performance, feedback, and assessment results.Recognizing successful training elements enables trainers to replicate effective strategies in future sessions, while addressing weaknesses helps refine and enhance the training program.

Making Targeted Adjustments - Based on evaluation findings, trainers can make targeted adjustments to training content, delivery methods, and instructional techniques to better meet participants' learning needs and preferences.

Adjustments may include revising curriculum materials, incorporating additional interactive activities, or providing supplementary resources to enhance learning outcomes.

PART FIVE

CASE STUDIES AND PRACTICAL SCENARIOS

Introduction.

Presented below are authentic case studies depicting incidents that have exerted substantial influence on the safeguarding sector. These examples are routinely incorporated into my training sessions to underscore the pervasive relevance of safeguarding principles in various spheres of daily existence.

Accompanying each case study are sets of discussion questions tailored for group engagement during training sessions. It's important to acknowledge that these scenarios reflect real events, some of which may elicit emotional responses from trainees. Thus, it's imperative to exercise sensitivity when integrating them into training sessions and to prioritise the well-being of participants. Additionally, remember to prioritise your own self-care and allow ample time for reflection following discussions of potentially distressing material.

<u>**Case Study 1 - The Shropshire Enquiry**</u>

The Shropshire Enquiry of 1945 marks a pivotal moment in the evolution of modern safeguarding practices in the United Kingdom. At its heart is the case of Dennis O'Niel, a 12-year-old boy whose plight thrust child protection into the national spotlight.

The tragic case of Dennis O'Neill, a 12-year-old boy from Newport, Monmouthshire, stands as a sobering reminder of the profound implications of safeguarding failures. On 30th May 1944, Dennis and his younger brothers, Terence and Frederick, were placed under the care of the Newport County Borough Council by the Newport Juvenile Court due to their need for care and attention. Subsequently, on 5th July 1944, Dennis and Terence were sent to live with Reginald and Esther Gough at their remote farm, Bank Farm, in the Hope Valley near Minsterley, Shropshire, England. Frederick was placed with a nearby couple, Mr. and Mrs. Pickering.

On 9th January 1945, Esther Gough called the local doctor to report that Dennis was experiencing a fit. When the doctor arrived, he found Dennis already deceased, in a severely malnourished and neglected state. An inquest determined that Dennis died of cardiac failure due to severe chest trauma and beating, coupled with chronic undernourishment and neglect. Reginald Gough was charged with manslaughter, while Esther Gough faced charges of wilful ill-treatment, neglect, and exposure likely to cause suffering and injury. Ultimately, Reginald Gough was convicted of manslaughter and sentenced to six years in prison, while Esther Gough received a six-month sentence for neglect.

The harrowing details of Dennis O'Neill's case shocked both the public and policymakers, prompting calls for inquiries and reforms in safeguarding practices. The case underscored the critical need for robust measures to protect vulnerable children and prevent such tragedies from recurring. As a result, the Home Secretary announced a public inquiry, chaired by Sir Walter Monckton, which identified systemic failures in safeguarding processes. Additionally, Shropshire County Council initiated its inquiry, highlighting the need for reorganisation in the boarding-out of children and stricter regulations for foster care.

The aftermath of Dennis O'Neill's case led to significant legislative changes, including the implementation of new regulations on the boarding-out of children. These regulations mandated the appointment of boarding-out committees, regular visits and medical examinations for foster children, and stringent vetting of foster parents. Furthermore, the case played a pivotal role in shaping the Curtis Report of 1946 and the subsequent Children Act of 1948, which sought to strengthen safeguarding provisions and protect the welfare of children across the UK.

Beyond its legal and legislative implications, the case of Dennis O'Neill has left an indelible mark on literature and popular culture. Agatha Christie's radio play "Three Blind Mice," inspired by the case, later evolved into the iconic stage play "The Mousetrap." Moreover, Terry O'Neill's non-fiction book, "Someone to Love Us," serves as a poignant reminder of the enduring legacy of Dennis O'Neill's tragic story and its profound impact on safeguarding practices in the UK.

Group discussion questions:

1 - What were the key failures in the safeguarding process that led to Dennis O'Neill's tragic death?

2 - How might the initial assessment and placement process have been improved to prevent such an outcome?

3 - What lessons can be learned from this case in terms of identifying and addressing safeguarding concerns within foster care and residential settings?

4 - How can professionals in various sectors collaborate more effectively to ensure the safety and protection of vulnerable children?

5 - What role does public awareness and advocacy play in holding institutions and authorities accountable for safeguarding failures?

6 - How can historical cases like Dennis O'Neill's inform current safeguarding practices and policies?

7 - What steps can be taken to promote a culture of transparency, accountability, and continuous improvement in safeguarding systems and procedures?

<u>**Case Study 2 - Victoria Climbie**</u>

Victoria Climbié was born on 2 November 1991 in Abobo, Ivory Coast, as the fifth child among seven siblings to Francis Climbié and Berthe Amoissi. Her aunt, Marie-Thérèse Kouao, who lived in France with her three sons, visited the Climbié family in October 1998, expressing her desire to take a child back to France for education, a common practice in their society. Victoria's parents, although having met Kouao only a few times, agreed to the arrangement, and Victoria was chosen for the journey.

Kouao falsely claimed Victoria as her daughter and gave her the name Anna, using a false passport to travel to Europe. Victoria, now known as Anna, and Kouao initially settled in Paris, France, but soon moved to the United Kingdom in April - June 1999, where they lived in various locations in London. Despite numerous opportunities for intervention, Victoria's welfare was severely neglected. She suffered abuse and neglect while under the care of Kouao and her partner, Carl Manning. The authorities were alerted to Victoria's situation on multiple occasions, but inadequate responses and missed opportunities allowed the abuse to continue. In July 1999, Victoria was admitted to the Central Middlesex Hospital with severe injuries, but misdiagnosis and failures in the child protection system resulted in her being discharged back into the care of Kouao and Manning.

On 7 August 1999, Kouao went to Ealing social services, but they dismissed her concerns about housing, deeming it a closed case. 6 days later, a consultant Doctor at Central Middlesex hospital wrote to Brent council, asking them to look into Victoria's case. However, there was confusion about whether communication occurred between social workers. Despite subsequent letters and discussions, no concrete action was taken. A social worker visited Victoria's home twice, but failed to detect any signs of abuse.

Kouao began avoiding hospitals and turned to churches, claiming Victoria was possessed by demons. Pastors attempted to exorcise the supposed demons, attributing Victoria's injuries to possession. Manning subjected Victoria to horrific abuse, forcing her to sleep in a bathtub filled with her own waste from October 1999 to January 2000.

Victoria's deteriorating condition was tragically overlooked until 24 February 2000 when she was rushed to the hospital in critical condition. Despite efforts to save her, Victoria sadly passed away the following day. A postmortem revealed 128 injuries, highlighting the severity of the abuse she endured.

Kouao and Manning were arrested shortly after Victoria's death and stood trial for child cruelty and murder. Manning admitted to cruelty and manslaughter, while Kouao denied all charges. Both were found guilty on 12 January 2001 and sentenced to life imprisonment. The judge condemned their actions, describing Victoria's suffering as unimaginable and holding them responsible for her tragic death.

Victoria's death prompted significant reforms in child protection policies and practices in the United Kingdom, including the introduction of the Children Act 2004 and the establishment of initiatives such as Every Child Matters and the Office of the Children's Commissioner. Her case serves as a sobering reminder of the importance of effective safeguarding measures and the need for vigilance in protecting vulnerable children from harm.

Group discussion questions:

1 - Discuss the warning signs of abuse and neglect that were present in Victoria Climbié's case. How could these signs have been recognized earlier by the various agencies involved?

2 - Explore the communication breakdowns between different agencies, such as social services, healthcare providers, and law enforcement, in Victoria's case. What measures can be implemented to improve communication and information sharing?

3 - Consider the role of training and awareness-raising initiatives in preventing similar cases of child abuse and neglect. How can frontline workers be better equipped to recognize and respond to signs of abuse?

4 - Identify the lessons learned from Victoria's case and discuss the systemic changes that have been implemented since her death to improve child protection services.

5 - Explore the support services available for victims and survivors of child abuse and neglect. How can these services be improved to better meet the needs of vulnerable individuals?

6 - Brainstorm prevention strategies to identify and address child abuse and neglect at an early stage. How can communities work together to create safer environments for children?

<u>**Case Study 3 - Steven Hoskin**</u>

Steven Hoskin was a vulnerable adult who lived in St. Austell, Cornwall, United Kingdom. He had a learning disability and mental health issues, which made him particularly susceptible to exploitation and abuse. Steven had a troubled upbringing and had spent much of his life in and out of care facilities.

Steven's perpetrators were a group of individuals who befriended him under the guise of friendship but ultimately subjected him to horrific abuse and ultimately led to his death. Among them were Sarah Bullock, Darren Stewart, and three others. Bullock had a history of violence and was known to manipulate vulnerable individuals for her own gain. Steven initially met Bullock and Stewart in the summer of 2005. They portrayed themselves as friends and gained his trust, exploiting his vulnerabilities for financial gain.

As their relationship with Steven deepened, Bullock and Stewart isolated him from his family and friends, exerting control over his life. They manipulated him into signing over his benefits and took control of his finances. Bullock and Stewart subjected Steven to severe physical and psychological abuse, including beatings, humiliation, and forced ingestion of drugs and alcohol. They used fear and intimidation to maintain control over him.

Steven was coerced into participating in criminal activities, including theft and drug dealing, by Bullock and Stewart. He was threatened with violence if he refused to comply with their demands. On July 6, 2006, Steven was subjected to a particularly brutal attack orchestrated by Bullock, Stewart, and their associates. He was brutally beaten, bound with tape, and taken to a viaduct where he was thrown off to his death. His body was found the next day.

Despite Steven's vulnerability and the signs of abuse, there were missed opportunities for intervention by social services, healthcare professionals, and law enforcement agencies. Concerns raised by Steven's family and support workers were not adequately addressed. Various agencies failed to recognize the warning signs of abuse, including Steven's unexplained injuries, changes in behaviour, and financial exploitation. There was a lack of coordination and communication between different services involved in his care.

Steven did not receive adequate support and protection from the authorities, leaving him vulnerable to further abuse and exploitation. There was a failure to implement safeguarding measures and provide him with the necessary support to escape his abusive situation.

The death of Steven Hoskin serves as a tragic reminder of the vulnerabilities faced by individuals with learning disabilities and mental health issues. It highlights the importance of robust safeguarding measures and effective intervention strategies to protect vulnerable adults from abuse and exploitation.

Group discussion questions:

1 - Discuss the characteristics and circumstances that make individuals like Steven Hoskin vulnerable to abuse and exploitation. Explore how to recognize signs of vulnerability and the importance of early intervention to prevent harm.

2 - Explore the indicators of abuse and exploitation in vulnerable adults, including physical injuries, changes in behaviour, and financial exploitation. Discuss the importance of thorough assessments and regular monitoring to identify and respond to signs of abuse promptly.

3 - Review the process of conducting risk assessments for vulnerable adults and developing tailored support plans to mitigate risks. Discuss strategies for managing risks associated with exploitation, including safeguarding measures and crisis intervention protocols.

4 - Explore ways to empower vulnerable adults to assert their rights and seek help if they experience abuse or exploitation. Discuss the role of advocacy support, accessible reporting mechanisms, and education in promoting self-advocacy and autonomy.

5 - Consider the impact of cultural factors, cognitive abilities, and diverse backgrounds on safeguarding vulnerable adults. Discuss strategies for promoting cultural competence, addressing intersectional vulnerabilities, and ensuring inclusive safeguarding practices.

6 - Encourage participants to reflect on their own attitudes, biases, and practices related to safeguarding vulnerable adults. Discuss the importance of ongoing training, supervision, and self-awareness in enhancing professional practice and promoting effective safeguarding outcomes.

<u>**Case Study 4 - Banaz Mahmod**</u>

Banaz Mahmod was a 20-year-old British Iraqi Kurdish woman who became the victim of an honor killing orchestrated by her family members in 2006. Her tragic death highlights significant failures in safeguarding and protecting vulnerable individuals from so-called "honour-based violence."

Banaz Mahmod was born in Iraq in 1985 but later moved to the United Kingdom as a child refugee fleeing the regime of Saddam Hussein. Growing up in London, she faced cultural clashes between the conservative beliefs of her family and her desire for independence and freedom. Banaz sought to break free from her family's strict control and pursue a relationship with a man of her own choice, which led to conflict and tension within her family.

In 2005, Banaz reported to the police that she was being threatened by members of her family due to her relationship. She expressed fears for her safety and provided detailed information about the threats she faced, including the names of individuals involved. Despite her courageous efforts to seek help, Banaz's case was not treated with the seriousness and urgency it deserved.

Tragically, Banaz's worst fears were realised when she was brutally murdered by members of her own family in January 2006. Her body was found buried in a suitcase in a backyard in Birmingham, showing signs of torture and violence. It was later revealed that Banaz had been raped, strangled, and subjected to horrific abuse before her death.

The investigation into Banaz's murder uncovered shocking revelations about the extent of the abuse she suffered at the hands of her family. She had been subjected to repeated acts of violence, including being raped and assaulted, in an attempt to control her behavior and enforce their twisted concept of honor. Despite her pleas for help and attempts to escape the abuse, Banaz was failed by the authorities who did not take adequate action to protect her.

Her father, Mahmod Mahmod, and uncle, Ari Mahmod, were among those convicted of orchestrating and carrying out the murder. Others involved included individuals from the Kurdish community who assisted in the planning and execution of the crime. The trial revealed the extent of the conspiracy and the roles played by each perpetrator in the brutal killing of Banaz Mahmod.

The case sparked widespread outrage and prompted a national inquiry into honour-based violence and forced marriage in the UK. It shed light on the challenges faced by victims of such crimes in seeking help and protection from the authorities.

Group discussion questions:

1 - Discuss what honour-based violence is, its cultural contexts, and how it manifests in various forms of abuse, including forced marriages, honour killings, and other coercive control tactics.

2 - Explore the red flags and indicators that someone may be at risk of honour-based violence or forced marriage. This could include signs of isolation, withdrawal, changes in behaviour, or expressions of fear.

3 - Discuss the cultural, social, and familial barriers that may prevent victims from seeking help or reporting abuse. Explore strategies for overcoming these barriers and creating safe spaces for disclosure.

4 - Emphasise the need for cultural competence and sensitivity when working with individuals from diverse backgrounds. Discuss how cultural beliefs and norms may impact perceptions of abuse and influence help-seeking behaviours.

5 - Explore the specific support needs of survivors of honour-based violence and forced marriage. Discuss trauma-informed approaches to service provision, access to culturally appropriate support services, and the importance of survivor-centred advocacy.

6 - Discuss strategies for preventing honour-based violence and forced marriage, including community outreach and education, awareness campaigns, and early intervention initiatives.

APPENDIX 1

SELF-CARE AND PERSONAL WELLBEING

Introduction

In the realm of safeguarding, where the responsibilities are weighty and the stakes are high, it's easy for safeguarding leads to become so engrossed in their roles that they neglect their own self-care and personal wellbeing. However, it's imperative to recognize that safeguarding work can be emotionally and mentally demanding, often exposing individuals to distressing situations and traumatic experiences. Therefore, this section of the manual aims to remind safeguarding leads of the critical importance of prioritising their own self-care and wellbeing. By maintaining a healthy balance between professional responsibilities and personal needs, safeguarding leads can sustain their effectiveness, resilience, and overall wellbeing while fulfilling their vital role in protecting vulnerable individuals and communities.

Recognizing and addressing the emotional impact of safeguarding work is essential for safeguarding leads to effectively fulfil their roles and maintain their wellbeing. Safeguarding leads often encounter distressing and emotionally challenging situations while working with vulnerable individuals who have experienced abuse, neglect, or exploitation. Witnessing or hearing about these traumatic experiences can evoke a range of emotions, including sadness, anger, frustration, and helplessness. Moreover, safeguarding leads may feel overwhelmed by the responsibility of advocating for and protecting those in vulnerable situations, especially when faced with systemic barriers or limitations.

The emotional toll of safeguarding work can manifest in various ways, both personally and professionally. Safeguarding leads may experience increased stress levels, difficulty sleeping, irritability, and a sense of emotional exhaustion. Furthermore, repeatedly engaging with traumatic stories and situations can lead to compassion fatigue or vicarious trauma, where individuals experience symptoms similar to those of individuals directly exposed to trauma. It's crucial for safeguarding leads to recognize these signs and acknowledge the impact that their work may have on their emotional wellbeing.

To address the emotional impact of safeguarding work, safeguarding leads must prioritize self-awareness and self-care. This involves regularly checking in with oneself to assess emotional responses and recognizing when additional support or resources may be needed. Safeguarding leads should cultivate a supportive network of colleagues, supervisors, or mental health professionals whom they can turn to for guidance, debriefing, and emotional support. Creating a culture of open communication and psychological safety within the safeguarding team can also encourage individuals to share their experiences and seek assistance when necessary.

Additionally, safeguarding leads should engage in self-care practices that promote emotional resilience and wellbeing. This may include setting boundaries around work-related responsibilities, taking regular breaks to recharge, participating in hobbies or activities that bring joy, and practising mindfulness or relaxation techniques.

Tips for self care and managing burnout

Managing stress and preventing burnout is crucial for safeguarding leads to maintain their wellbeing and effectiveness in their role. Here is a practical list of strategies for managing stress and preventing burnout:

Set Boundaries - Establish clear boundaries between work and personal life. Allocate specific times for work-related tasks and ensure to disconnect and focus on personal activities during non-work hours.

Prioritise Tasks - Identify and prioritise tasks based on urgency and importance. Break down large tasks into smaller, manageable steps to prevent feeling overwhelmed.

Delegate Responsibility - Delegate tasks to other team members or colleagues when possible. Sharing responsibilities can alleviate workload pressure and promote a sense of teamwork.

Practice Self-Care - Engage in regular self-care activities such as exercise, meditation, hobbies, or spending time with loved ones. Prioritise activities that bring joy and relaxation to recharge your energy.

Seek Support - Build a supportive network of colleagues, mentors, or supervisors whom you can confide in and seek guidance from. Don't hesitate to reach out for support when needed.

Attend Training and Supervision - Participate in regular training sessions and supervision meetings to enhance skills, discuss challenging cases, and receive feedback. Continuous learning and professional development can boost confidence and resilience.

Set Realistic Expectations - Avoid setting unrealistic expectations for yourself or others. Recognize that you cannot solve every problem or prevent every adverse outcome, and focus on what you can control.

Practice Mindfulness - Incorporate mindfulness or relaxation techniques into your daily routine to manage stress and promote emotional wellbeing. Mindfulness practices such as deep breathing, meditation, or progressive muscle relaxation can help reduce tension and promote mental clarity.

Take Breaks - Take regular breaks throughout the day to rest and recharge. Stepping away from work, even for a short period, can help prevent burnout and improve productivity.

Monitor Stress Levels - Pay attention to your stress levels and recognize signs of burnout, such as feeling exhausted, irritable, or apathetic. Take proactive steps to address stressors and seek support if needed.

Celebrate Successes - Acknowledge and celebrate your achievements and successes, no matter how small. Recognizing your contributions and progress can boost morale and motivation.

By implementing these strategies and prioritising self-care, safeguarding leads can effectively manage stress, prevent burnout, and continue to fulfil their important role in protecting vulnerable individuals.

Afterword.

Thank you for reading this guide. I sincerely hope this helps new safeguarding leads to navigate their newly found responsibilities. And if you are not brand new, I hope this proves a valuable reference text.

I immensely enjoy my role as a safeguarding lead and I find it fascinating how the job constantly evolves and adapts to new changes and risks. I hope in the future that this book will also change and adapt with the times into future editions, remaining relevant and up to date.

Remember - Not everything rests on your shoulders. Utilize your colleagues. Don't be afraid to ask for help, advice, or just for someone to act as a sounding board. And always take time for your self-care. Keep reflecting and don't allow burnout to creep in.

Again, thank you for reading and making use of The New Safeguarding Lead.

Paul Armstrong
April 2024

www.ingramcontent.com/pod-product-compliance
Lightning Source LLC
Chambersburg PA
CBHW051102250726
48656CB00001B/426

9 798322 203810